MEDITERRANEAN DIE AND BUSY MAN DIET

TWO SIMPLE GUIDES ONE FOR FOLLOWING THE MEDITERRANEAN DIET AND ONE FOR THE BUSY MAN DIET, TOGETHER WITH TWO SPECIFIC COOKBOOKS TO PLAN THE TWO DIETS AND LOSE WEIGHT (250+RECIPES)

TWO BOOKS IN ONE

By

Lisa STAR

<u>AUTHOR'S NOTE</u>: Calorie indications are for one serve

This book has given you all the information you need to do this diet correctly and do it right. It is essential to understand what you are getting into when you embark on this diet, and this book gave you valuable information that you can use to your advantage and avoid the problems that can come with this diet. You want to stay healthy and make sure that your body can do what it needs to do. As with anything, we emphasize that if something seems wrong or unnatural, you will need to see a doctor to make sure you are safe and that your body can handle this diet. Use the knowledge in this book to get amazing recipes and learn directions for excellent meals for yourself. Consult your doctor before to starting new diet.

TABLE OF CONTENS

MEDITERRANEAN DIET

MEDITERRANEAN DIET
INTRODUCTION

MEDITERRANEAN CUISINE

The Mediterranean is a large region made up of many different countries, so people of the same nationality do not all eat the same foods, which shows that the benefits of this diet are not just due to certain foods. In fact, the benefits come from a particular diet and the foods together. It can greatly expand the types of foods you can eat, rather than leaving you with a limited list of foods. I will explain in more detail what the Mediterranean diet is and what you can eat (including things you should limit or avoid altogether). So bear in mind that all the information given is for guidance only and you can adapt the plans and recipes given to suit your own preferences. As with all diets, if you have any doubts or are taking medication, always consult your doctor before starting a diet.

EATING REGULARLY

Vegetables: cucumbers, carrots, cauliflower, tomatoes, broccoli, cabbage, onions, spinach and others.
Seeds and nuts: almonds, walnuts, sunflower, pumpkin, cashews, etc. Potatoes, turnips, sweet potatoes, etc.
Poultry: chicken, turkey or duck. Whole grains: whole-grain bread, pasta, barley, corn, brown rice, etc.
Note: In the Mediterranean, bread is generally only used for dipping, not for sandwiches. Herbs and spices: garlic, rosemary, sage, pepper, etc. Fish and crustaceans: mackerel, trout, salmon, shrimps, prawns, mussels, etc.
Fruit: apples, oranges, pears, figs, dates, avocados, berries and many more. Legumes: beans, peas, lentils, chickpeas, etc. Extra virgin olive oil and olives, avocado oil. Olive oil, olive oil, olive oil, olive oil, olive oil, olive oil, olive oil, olive oil, olive oil, olive oil.

MODERATE EATING

Yoghurt, cheese, poultry and eggs. Less consumption of red meat and red meat.

WHAT TO AVOID

Processed foods - low-fat, diet or convenience foods. Processed meat - hot dogs, sausages, etc.
Trans fatty acids - found in processed foods and margarine. Refined grains - all refined wheat products, white bread, pasta, etc. Refined oils - rapeseed oil, soybean oil, etc. Sweet - Sugar in tea, coffee, lemonade, cakes and ice cream.

DRINKS

Unlike most diets, coffee and tea are allowed, and one glass of red wine per day is recommended. Water should be drunk throughout the day to keep you hydrated and to help flush the body. Fruit juices and sugary drinks should be avoided as they contain extra sugar.

SNACKS

The Mediterranean way of eating usually involves only three meals a day, but if you are hungry between meals, here are some snacks: half a cup of nuts, half a cup of berries, raw carrots and fruit.

EATING THE MEDITERRANEAN DIET

If you eat in restaurants, you probably realise that this is one of the easiest diets to follow, so here are some tips on how to get your meals the right way. Order wholemeal bread and ask if olive oil is available instead of butter. Ask if they can fry your food in olive oil, or if you can have your food steamed. Choose fish or seafood as your main dish. The general advice is that your body should not use a quick fix or starve itself for certain foods needed for normal daily activities. The goal is to eat a healthy diet every day, with no side effects if followed for a long period of time as with some diets. In general, you should aim to maximise your intake of some of the foods listed in the 'eat often' section, such as fruit, vegetables, pulses and berries.whole grains. Limit the amount of salt used in cooking, as an increase in salt is directly linked to high blood pressure. Alternatives to salt include herbs and spices and garlic. The main Mediterranean countries are Greece, Spain and southern Italy. Once you have seen and tried some of the recipes in this book, it is easy to find other healthy alternatives from these countries. You will soon discover that with a little modification they can easily be incorporated into your diet, as most of the recipes are already dietary. You will also notice that the recipes include a high consumption of legumes, which are recommended on a regular basis along with unrefined cereals, fruits and vegetables, especially green leafy ones. They all use a lot of olive oil, both for cooking and seasoning. Also note that most recipes call for fish or seafood and recommend them in place of poultry and red meat. Many studies have shown that the main contributor to the benefits of a diet is actually olive oil, and where possible you should aim to use extra virgin olive oil. And although it is slightly more expensive, it is of much higher quality - in fact, it is the purest oil obtained from the first pressing of the olives. It has been said that olive oil can reduce the risk of all types of cancer, cardiovascular disease and other chronic illnesses. Although there are many countries in the Mediterranean region, this diet takes a broad look at the foods and recipes available in all these countries and many others. I have tried not to limit the recipes to a specific country. Also note that you can drink 2 small glasses of red wine or 1 large glass a day, and studies show that this alone can help reduce the risk of heart disease, stroke, diabetes and premature death. Note that drinking large amounts can actually increase the risk of diseases that small amounts help treat. Although this diet has been known for years, the Barcelona Mediterranean Diet Foundation continues to research the benefits of the Mediterranean diet. It is also important to note that their aim is to promote research into the health, historical, cultural and gastronomic aspects of the Mediterranean diet. In addition to their own studies, they analyse the scientific results of tests carried out by others, in accordance with regulatory guidelines. It shows how important it is that

NOTE: This book has given you all the information you need to do this diet correctly and do it right. It is essential to understand what you are getting into when you embark on this diet, and this book gave you valuable information that you can use to your advantage and avoid the problems that can come with this diet. You want to stay healthy and make sure that your body can do what it needs to do. As with anything, we emphasize that if something seems wrong or unnatural, you will need to see a doctor to make sure you are safe and that your body can handle this diet. Use the knowledge in this book to get amazing recipes and learn directions for excellent meals for yourself. Consult your doctor before to starting new diet.

1. ROAST ASPARAGUS

Servings: 4 **Cook Time: 5 Min** **Prep Time 15 Min**

INGREDIENTS:

- ✓ 1 tbsp Extra virgin olive oil (1 tablespoon)
- ✓ 1 medium lemon
- ✓ ½ tsp Freshly grated nutmeg
- ✓ ½ tsp black pepper
- ✓ ½ tsp Kosher salt

DIRECTIONS:

- ➢ Warm the oven to 500°F
- ➢ Put the asparagus on an aluminum foil
- ➢ Drizzle with extra virgin olive oil, and toss until well coated.
- ➢ Roast the asparagus in the oven for about five minutes
- ➢ Toss and continue roasting until browned
- ➢ Sprinkle the roasted asparagus with nutmeg, salt, zest, and pepper.

NUTRITION INFORMATION: Calories: 123 Carbs: 5g Fat: 11g Protein: 3g

2. FISH FILLET ON LEMONS

Servings: 4 **Cook Time: 6 Min** **Prep Time 5 Min**

INGREDIENTS:

- ✓ 4 (4-ounce/ 113-g) fish fillets, such as tilapia, salmon, catfish, cod, or your favorite fish
- ✓ Nonstick cooking spray
- ✓ 3 to 4 medium lemons
- ✓ 1 tablespoon extra-virgin olive oil
- ✓ ¼ teaspoon freshly ground black pepper
- ✓ ¼ teaspoon kosher or sea salt

DIRECTIONS:

- ➢ Use paper towels, pat the fillets dry and let stand at room temperature for 10 minutes
- ➢ Meanwhile, coat the cold cooking grate of the grill with nonstick cooking spray
- ➢ Preheat the grill to 400°F (205°C), or medium-high heat
- ➢ Or preheat a grill pan over medium-high heat on the stove top.
- ➢ Cut one lemon in half and set half aside
- ➢ Slice the remaining half of that lemon and the remaining lemons into ¼-inch-thick slices
- ➢ (You should have about 12 to 16 lemon slices.)
- ➢ Into a small bowl, squeeze 1 tablespoon of juice out of the reserved lemon half.
- ➢ Add the oil to the bowl with the lemon juice
- ➢ Mix well. Brush both sides of the fish with the oil mixture
- ➢ Sprinkle evenly with pepper and salt.
- ➢ Carefully place the lemon slices on the grill (or the grill pan)
- ➢ Arrange 3 to 4 slices together in the shape of a fish fillet
- ➢ Repeat with the remaining slices
- ➢ Place the fish fillets directly on top of the lemon slices
- ➢ Grill with the lid closed
- ➢ (If you're grilling on the stove top, cover with a large pot lid or aluminum foil.)
- ➢ Turn the fish halfway through the cooking time
- ➢ (Only if the fillets are more than half an inch thick)
- ➢ The fish is done and ready to serve
- ➢ (When it just begins to separate into flakes (chunks) when pressed gently with a fork).

NUTRITION INFORMATION: Calories: 208 fat: 11g protein: 21g carbs: 2g fiber: 0g sodium: 249mg

3. PANKO-CRUSTED FISH STICKS

Servings: 4   **Cook Time: 5 Min**   **Prep Time 10 Min**

INGREDIENTS:

- ✓ 2 large eggs, lightly beaten
- ✓ 1 tablespoon 2% milk
- ✓ 1 pound (454 g) skinned fish fillets (cod, tilapia, or other white fish) about ½ inch thick, sliced into 20 (1-inch-wide) strips
- ✓ ½ cup yellow cornmeal
- ✓ ½ cup whole-wheat panko bread crumbs or whole-wheat bread crumbs
- ✓ ¼ teaspoon smoked paprika
- ✓ ¼ teaspoon kosher or sea salt
- ✓ ¼ teaspoon freshly ground black pepper
- ✓ Nonstick cooking spray

DIRECTIONS:

- ➢ Place a large, rimmed baking sheet in the oven
- ➢ Preheat the oven to 400°F (205°C) with the pan inside.
- ➢ In a large bowl, mix the eggs and milk
- ➢ Use a fork, add the fish strips to the egg mixture and stir gently to coat
- ➢ Put the cornmeal, bread crumbs
- ➢ Add smoked paprika, salt, and pepper in a quart-size zip-top plastic bag
- ➢ Use a fork or tongs, transfer the fish to the bag
- ➢ Let the excess egg wash drip off into the bowl before transferring
- ➢ Seal the bag and shake gently to completely coat each fish stick.
- ➢ With oven mitts, carefully remove the hot baking sheet from the oven
- ➢ Spray it with nonstick cooking spray
- ➢ Use a fork or tongs, remove the fish sticks from the bag
- ➢ Arrange them on the hot baking sheet, with space between them
- ➢ (So the hot air can circulate and crisp them up)
- ➢ Bake for 5 to 8 minutes
- ➢ (Until gentle pressure with a fork causes the fish to flake)
- ➢ Serve.

NUTRITION INFORMATION: Calories: 238 fat: 2g protein: 22g carbs: 28g fiber: 1g sodium: 494mg

4. OREGANO SHRIMP PUTTANESCA

Servings: 4   **Cook Time: 9 Min**   **Prep Time 10 Min**

INGREDIENTS:

- ✓ 2 tablespoons extra-virgin olive oil
- ✓ 3 anchovy fillets, drained and chopped, or 1½ teaspoons anchovy paste
- ✓ 3 garlic cloves, minced
- ✓ ½ teaspoon crushed red pepper
- ✓ 1 (14½-ounce / 411-g) can low-sodium or no-salt-added diced tomatoes, undrained
- ✓ 1 (2¼-ounce / 64-g) can sliced black olives, drained
- ✓ 2 tablespoons capers
- ✓ 1 tablespoon chopped fresh oregano or
- ✓ 1 teaspoon dried oregano
- ✓ 1 pound fresh raw shrimp (or frozen and thawed shrimp), shells and tails removed

DIRECTIONS:

- ➢ In a large skillet over medium heat, heat the oil
- ➢ Mix in the anchovies, garlic, and crushed red pepper
- ➢ Cook for 3 minutes, stirring frequently and mashing up the anchovies with a wooden spoon
- ➢ (Until they have melted into the oil)
- ➢ Stir in the tomatoes with their juices, olives, capers, and oregano
- ➢ Turn up the heat to medium-high, and bring to a simmer.
- ➢ When the sauce is lightly bubbling, stir in the shrimp
- ➢ Reduce the heat to medium
- ➢ Cook the shrimp for 6 to 8 minutes
- ➢ (Or until they turn pink and white, stirring occasionally)
- ➢ Serve.

NUTRITION INFORMATION: Calories: 362 fat: 12g protein: 30g carbs: 31g fiber: 1g sodium: 1463mg

5. SICILIAN TUNA AND VEGGIE BOWL

Servings: 6   **Cook Time: 16 Min**   **Prep Time 10 Min**

INGREDIENTS:

- ✓ 1 pound (454 g) kale, chopped, center ribs removed
- ✓ 3 tablespoons extra-virgin olive oil
- ✓ 1 cup chopped onion
- ✓ 3 garlic cloves, minced
- ✓ 1 (2¼-ounce / 64-g) can sliced olives, drained
- ✓ ¼ cup capers
- ✓ ¼ teaspoon crushed red pepper
- ✓ 2 teaspoons sugar
- ✓ 2 (6-ounce / 170-g) cans tuna in olive oil, undrained
- ✓ 1 (15-ounce / 425-g) can cannellini beans or great northern beans, drained and rinsed
- ✓ ¼ teaspoon freshly ground black pepper
- ✓ ¼ teaspoon kosher or sea salt

DIRECTIONS:

- ➢ Fill a large stockpot three-quarters full of water, and bring to a boil
- ➢ Add the kale and cook for 2 minutes
- ➢ (This is to make the kale less bitter.)
- ➢ Drain the kale in a colander and set aside.
- ➢ Set the empty pot back on the stove over medium heat
- ➢ Pour in the oil. Add the onion and cook for 4 minutes, stirring often
- ➢ Then the garlic and cook for 1 minute, stirring often
- ➢ Join also the olives, capers, and crushed red pepper
- ➢ Cook for 1 minute, stirring often. Add the partially cooked kale and sugar
- ➢ Stir until the kale is completely coated with oil
- ➢ Cover the pot and cook for 8 minutes.
- ➢ Remove the kale from the heat, mix in the tuna, beans, pepper, and salt
- ➢ Serve.

NUTRITION INFORMATION: Calories: 372 | fat: 28g | protein: 8g | carbs: 22g | fiber: 7g | sodium: 452mg:

6. SEA BASS WITH ROASTED ROOT VEGGIE

Servings: 15   **Cook Time: 15 Min**   **Prep Time 10 Min**

INGREDIENTS:

- ✓ 1 carrot, diced small 1 parsnip, diced small
- ✓ 1 rutabaga, diced small
- ✓ ¼ cup olive oil
- ✓ 2 teaspoons salt, divided
- ✓ 4 sea bass fillets
- ✓ ½ teaspoon onion powder
- ✓ 2 garlic cloves, minced
- ✓ 1 lemon, sliced, plus additional wedges for serving

DIRECTIONS:

- ➢ Preheat the air fryer to 380°F (193°C).
- ➢ In a small bowl, toss the carrot, parsnip, and rutabaga with olive oil and 1 teaspoon salt.
- ➢ Lightly season the sea bass with the remaining 1 teaspoon of salt and the onion powder
- ➢ Then place it into the air fryer basket in a single layer.
- ➢ Spread the garlic over the top of each fillet, then cover with lemon slices.
- ➢ Pour the prepared vegetables into the basket around and on top of the fish
- ➢ Roast for 15 minutes.
- ➢ Serve with additional lemon wedges if desired.

NUTRITION INFORMATION: Calories: 299 fat: 15g protein: 25g carbs: 13g fiber: 2g sodium: 1232mg

7. SHRIMP AND VEGGIE PITA

Servings: 4   **Cook Time: 6 Min**   **Prep Time 15 Min**

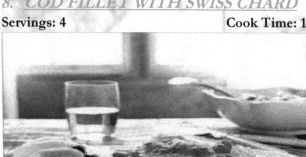

INGREDIENTS:

- ✓ 1 pound (454 g) medium shrimp, peeled and deveined
- ✓ 2 tablespoons olive oil
- ✓ 1 teaspoon dried oregano
- ✓ ½ teaspoon dried thyme
- ✓ ½ teaspoon garlic powder
- ✓ ¼ teaspoon onion powder
- ✓ ½ teaspoon salt
- ✓ ¼ teaspoon black pepper
- ✓ 4 whole wheat pitas
- ✓ 4 ounces (113 g) feta cheese, crumbled
- ✓ 1 cup shredded lettuce
- ✓ 1 tomato, diced
- ✓ ¼ cup black olives, sliced
- ✓ 1 lemon

DIRECTIONS:

- ➢ Preheat the oven to 380ºF (193ºC).
- ➢ In a medium bowl, combine the shrimp with the olive oil, oregano
- ➢ Add thyme, garlic powder, onion powder, salt, and black pepper.
- ➢ Pour shrimp in a single layer in the air fryer basket
- ➢ Cook for 6 to 8 minutes, or until cooked through.
- ➢ Remove from the air fryer
- ➢ Divide into warmed pitas with feta, lettuce, tomato, olives
- ➢ Than squeeze of lemon.

NUTRITION INFORMATION: Calories: 395 fat: 15g protein: 26g carbs: 40g fiber: 4g sodium: 728mg

8. COD FILLET WITH SWISS CHARD

Servings: 4   **Cook Time: 12 Min**   **Prep Time 10 Min**

INGREDIENTS:

- ✓ 1 teaspoon salt
- ✓ ½ teaspoon dried oregano
- ✓ ½ teaspoon dried thyme
- ✓ ½ teaspoon garlic powder
- ✓ 4 cod fillets
- ✓ ½ white onion, thinly sliced
- ✓ 2 cups Swiss chard, washed, stemmed, and torn into pieces
- ✓ ¼ cup olive oil
- ✓ 1 lemon, quartered

DIRECTIONS:

- ➢ Preheat the air fryer to 380ºF (193ºC).
- ➢ In a small bowl, whisk together the salt, oregano, thyme, and garlic powder.
- ➢ Tear off four pieces of aluminum foil, with each sheet being large enough to envelop one cod fillet and a quarter of the vegetables.
- ➢ Place a cod fillet in the middle of each sheet of foil
- ➢ Then sprinkle on all sides with the spice mixture.
- ➢ In each foil packet, place a quarter of the onion slices and ½ cup Swiss chard
- ➢ Then drizzle 1 tablespoon olive oil and squeeze ¼ lemon over the contents of each foil packet.
- ➢ Fold and seal the sides of the foil packets
- ➢ Then place them into the air fryer basket. Steam for 12 minutes.
- ➢ Remove from the basket, and carefully open each packet to avoid a steam burn.

NUTRITION INFORMATION: Calories: 252 fat: 13g protein: 26g carbs: 4g fiber: 1g sodium: 641mg

9. POLLOCK AND VEGETABLE PITAS

Servings: 4   **Cook Time: 15 Min**   **Prep Time 10 Min**

INGREDIENTS:

- ✓ 1 pound (454 g) pollock, cut into
- ✓ 1-inch pieces
- ✓ ¼ cup olive oil
- ✓ 1 teaspoon salt
- ✓ ½ teaspoon dried oregano
- ✓ ½ teaspoon dried thyme
- ✓ ½ teaspoon garlic powder
- ✓ ¼ teaspoon cayenne 4 whole wheat pitas
- ✓ 1 cup shredded lettuce
- ✓ 2 Roma tomatoes, diced
- ✓ Nonfat plain Greek yogurt
- ✓ Lemon, quartered

DIRECTIONS:

- ➢ Preheat the air fryer to 380°F (193°C).
- ➢ In a medium bowl, combine the pollock with olive oil, salt, oregano, thyme, garlic powder, and cayenne.
- ➢ Put the pollock into the air fryer basket and cook for 15 minutes.
- ➢ Serve inside pitas with lettuce, tomato, and Greek yogurt with a lemon wedge on the side.

NUTRITION INFORMATION: Calories: 368 fat: 1g protein: 21g carbs: 38g fiber: 5g sodium: 514mg

10. DILL AND GARLIC STUFFED RED SNAPPER

Servings: 4   **Cook Time: 35 Min**   **Prep Time 10 Min**

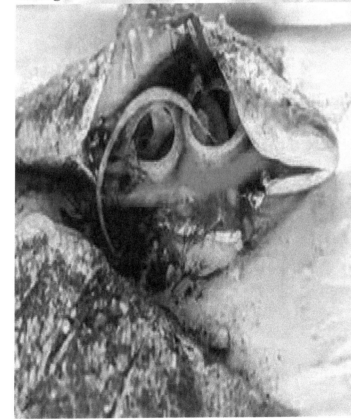

INGREDIENTS:

- ✓ 1 teaspoon salt
- ✓ ½ teaspoon black pepper
- ✓ ½ teaspoon ground cumin
- ✓ ¼ teaspoon cayenne
- ✓ 1 (1- to 1½-pound / 454- to 680-g) whole red snapper, cleaned and patted dry
- ✓ 2 tablespoons olive oil
- ✓ 2 garlic cloves, minced
- ✓ ¼ cup fresh dill
- ✓ Lemon wedges, for serving

DIRECTIONS:

- ➢ Preheat the air fryer to 360°F (182°C)
- ➢ In a small bowl, mix together the salt, pepper, cumin, and cayenne.
- ➢ Coat the outside of the fish with olive oil
- ➢ Then sprinkle the seasoning blend over the outside of the fish
- ➢ Stuff the minced garlic and dill inside the cavity of the fish.
- ➢ Place the snapper into the basket of the air fryer and roast for 20 minutes
- ➢ Flip the snapper over, and roast for 15 minutes more
- ➢ (Or until the snapper reaches an internal temperature of 145°F (63°C))

NUTRITION INFORMATION: Calories: 125 fat: 1g protein: 23g carbs: 2g fiber: 0g sodium: 562mg

11. EASY TUNA STEAKS

Servings: 4   **Cook Time: 8 Min**   **Prep Time 10 Min**

INGREDIENTS:

- ✓ 1 teaspoon garlic powder
- ✓ ½ teaspoon salt
- ✓ ¼ teaspoon dried thyme
- ✓ ¼ teaspoon dried oregano
- ✓ 4 tuna steaks
- ✓ 2 tablespoons olive oil
- ✓ 1 lemon, quartered

DIRECTIONS:

- ➢ Preheat the air fryer to 380°F (193°C).
- ➢ In a small bowl, whisk together the garlic powder, salt, thyme, and oregano.
- ➢ Coat the tuna steaks with olive oil
- ➢ Season both sides of each steak with the seasoning blend
- ➢ Place the steaks in a single layer in the air fryer basket.
- ➢ Cook for 5 minutes, then flip and cook for an additional 3 to 4 minutes.

NUTRITION INFORMATION: Calories: 269 fat: 13g protein: 33g carbs: 1g fiber: 0g sodium: 231mg

12. GREEK-STYLE LAMB BURGERS

Servings: 4   **Cook Time: 10 Min**   **Prep Time 10 Min**

INGREDIENTS:

- ✓ 1 pound (454 g) ground lamb
- ✓ ½ teaspoon salt
- ✓ ½ teaspoon freshly ground black pepper
- ✓ 4 tablespoons feta cheese, crumbled
- ✓ Buns, toppings, and tzatziki, for serving (optional)

DIRECTIONS:

- ➢ Preheat a grill, grill pan, or lightly oiled skillet to high heat.
- ➢ In a large bowl, using your hands
- ➢ Combine the lamb with the salt and pepper.
- ➢ Divide the meat into 4 portions. Divide each portion in half to make a top and a bottom
- ➢ Flatten each half into a 3-inch circle
- ➢ Make a dent in the center of one of the halves and place 1 tablespoon of the feta cheese in the center
- ➢ Place the second half of the patty on top of the feta cheese
- ➢ Press down to close the 2 halves together, making it resemble a round burger.
- ➢ Cook the stuffed patty for 3 minutes on each side, for medium-well
- ➢ Serve on a bun with your favorite toppings and tzatziki sauce, if desired.

NUTRITION INFORMATION: Calories: 345 fat: 29g protein: 20g carbs: 1g fiber: 0g sodium: 462mg

13. BRAISED VEAL SHANKS

Servings: 4 **Cook Time: 2 H** **Prep Time 10 Min**

INGREDIENTS:

- ✓ 4 veal shanks, bone in
- ✓ ½ cup flour
- ✓ 4 tablespoons extra-virgin olive oil
- ✓ 1 large onion, chopped
- ✓ 5 cloves garlic, sliced
- ✓ 2 teaspoons salt
- ✓ 1 tablespoon fresh thyme
- ✓ 3 tablespoons tomato paste
- ✓ 6 cups water
- ✓ Cooked noodles, for serving (optional)

DIRECTIONS:

- ➤ Preheat the oven to 350°F (180°C).
- ➤ Dredge the veal shanks in the flour.
- ➤ Pour the olive oil into a large oven-safe pot or pan over medium heat
- ➤ Add the veal shanks
- ➤ Brown the veal on both sides, about 4 minutes each side
- ➤ Remove the veal from pot and set aside.
- ➤ Add the onion, garlic, salt, thyme, and tomato paste to the pan
- ➤ Cook for 3 to 4 minutes. Add the water, and stir to combine.
- ➤ Then the veal back to the pan, and bring to a simmer
- ➤ Cover the pan with a lid or foil and bake for 1 hour and 50 minutes
- ➤ Remove from the oven and serve with cooked noodles, if desired.

NUTRITION INFORMATION: Calories: 400 fat: 19g protein: 39g carbs: 18g fiber: 2g sodium: 1368mg

14. GRILLED BEEF KEBABS

Servings: 6 **Cook Time: 10 Min** **Prep Time 15 Min**

INGREDIENTS:

- ✓ 2 pounds (907 g) beef fillet
- ✓ 1½ teaspoons salt
- ✓ 1 teaspoon freshly ground black pepper
- ✓ ½ teaspoon ground allspice
- ✓ ½ teaspoon ground nutmeg
- ✓ ⅓ cup extra-virgin olive oil
- ✓ 1 large onion, cut into
- ✓ 8 quarters
- ✓ 1 large red bell pepper, cut into
- ✓ 1-inch cubes

DIRECTIONS:

- ➤ Preheat a grill, grill pan, or lightly oiled skillet to high heat.
- ➤ Cut the beef into 1-inch cubes and put them in a large bowl.
- ➤ In a small bowl, mix together the salt, black pepper, allspice, and nutmeg.
- ➤ Pour the olive oil over the beef and toss to coat the beef
- ➤ Then evenly sprinkle the seasoning over the beef and toss to coat all pieces.
- ➤ Skewer the beef, alternating every 1 or 2 pieces with a piece of onion or bell pepper.
- ➤ To cook, place the skewers on the grill or skillet, and turn every 2 to 3 minutes until all sides have cooked to desired
- ➤ (Doneness, 6 minutes for medium-rare, 8 minutes for well done)
- ➤ Serve warm.

NUTRITION INFORMATION: Calories: 485 fat: 36g protein: 35g carbs: 4g fiber: 1g sodium: 1453mg

15. MEDITERRANEAN GRILLED SKIRT STEAK

Servings: 4   **Cook Time: 10 Min**   **Prep Time 10 Min**

INGREDIENTS:

- ✓ 1 pound (454 g) skirt steak
- ✓ 1 teaspoon salt
- ✓ ½ teaspoon freshly ground black pepper
- ✓ 2 cups prepared hummus
- ✓ 1 tablespoon extra-virgin olive oil
- ✓ ½ cup pine nuts

DIRECTIONS:

- ➤ Preheat a grill, grill pan, or lightly oiled skillet to medium heat.
- ➤ Season both sides of the steak with salt and pepper.
- ➤ Cook the meat on each side for 3 to 5 minutes; 3 minutes for medium, and 5 minutes on each side for well done
- ➤ Let the meat rest for 5 minutes.
- ➤ Slice the meat into thin strips.
- ➤ Spread the hummus on a serving dish, and evenly distribute the beef on top of the hummus.
- ➤ In a small saucepan, over low heat, add the olive oil and pine nuts
- ➤ Toast them for 3 minutes, constantly stirring them with a spoon so that they don't burn.
- ➤ Spoon the pine nuts over the beef and serve.

NUTRITION INFORMATION: Calories: 602 fat: 41g protein: 42g carbs: 20g fiber: 8g sodium: 1141mg

16. BEEF KEFTA

Servings: 4   **Cook Time: 5 Min**   **Prep Time 10 Min**

INGREDIENTS:

- ✓ 1 medium onion
- ✓ ⅓ cup fresh Italian parsley
- ✓ 1 pound (454 g) ground beef

- ✓ ¼ teaspoon ground cumin
- ✓ ¼ teaspoon cinnamon
- ✓ 1 teaspoon salt
- ✓ ½ teaspoon freshly ground black pepper

DIRECTIONS:

- ➤ Preheat a grill or grill pan to high.
- ➤ Mince the onion and parsley in a food processor until finely chopped.
- ➤ In a large bowl, using your hands
- ➤ Combine the beef with the onion mix, ground cumin, cinnamon, salt, and pepper.

- ➤ Divide the meat into 6 portions. Form each portion into a flat oval.
- ➤ Place the patties on the grill or grill pan and cook for 3 minutes on each side.

NUTRITION INFORMATION: Calories: 203 fat: 10g protein: 24g carbs: 3g fiber: 1g sodium: 655mg

17. BEEF AND POTATOES WITH TAHINI SAUCE

Servings: 6 **Cook Time: 30 Min** **Prep Time 10 Min**

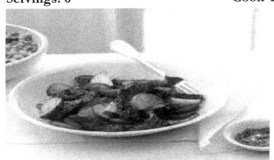

INGREDIENTS:

- ✓ 1 pound (454 g) ground beef
- ✓ 2 teaspoons salt, divided
- ✓ ½ teaspoon freshly ground black pepper
- ✓ 1 large onion, finely chopped
- ✓ 10 medium golden potatoes
- ✓ 2 tablespoons extra-virgin olive oil
- ✓ 3 cups Greek yogurt
- ✓ 1 cup tahini
- ✓ 3 cloves garlic, minced 2 cups water

DIRECTIONS:

- ➤ Preheat the oven to 450°F (235°C).
- ➤ In a large bowl, using your hands, combine the beef with 1 teaspoon salt, black pepper, and the onion.
- ➤ Form meatballs of medium size (about 1-inch), using about 2 tablespoons of the beef mixture
- ➤ Place them in a deep 8-by-8-inch casserole dish.
- ➤ Cut the potatoes into ¼-inch-thick slices
- ➤ Toss them with the olive oil.
- ➤ Lay the potato slices flat on a lined baking sheet.
- ➤ Put the baking sheet with the potatoes and the casserole dish with the meatballs in the oven
- ➤ Bake for 20 minutes.
- ➤ In a large bowl, mix together the yogurt, tahini, garlic, remaining 1 teaspoon salt, and water; set aside.

- ➤ Once you take the meatballs and potatoes out of the oven
- ➤ Use a spatula to transfer the potatoes from the baking sheet to the casserole dish with the meatballs
- ➤ Leave the beef drippings in the casserole dish for added flavor.
- ➤ Reduce the oven temperature to 375°F (190°C)
- ➤ Pour the yogurt tahini sauce over the beef and potatoes
- ➤ Return it to the oven for 10 minutes
- ➤ Once baking is complete, serve warm with a side of rice or pita bread.

NUTRITION INFORMATION: Calories: 1078 fat: 59g protein: 58g carbs: 89g fiber: 11g sodium: 1368mg

18. MEDITERRANEAN LAMB BOWLS

Servings: 2 **Cook Time: 15 Min** **Prep Time 15 Min**

INGREDIENTS:

- ✓ 2 tablespoons extra-virgin olive oil
- ✓ ¼ cup diced yellow onion
- ✓ 1 pound (454 g) ground lamb
- ✓ 1 teaspoon dried mint
- ✓ 1 teaspoon dried parsley
- ✓ ½ teaspoon red pepper flakes
- ✓ ¼ teaspoon garlic powder

- ✓ 1 cup cooked rice
- ✓ ½ teaspoon za'atar seasoning
- ✓ ½ cup halved cherry tomatoes
- ✓ 1 cucumber, peeled and diced
- ✓ 1 cup store-bought hummus
- ✓ 1 cup crumbled feta cheese
- ✓ 2 pita breads, warmed (optional)

DIRECTIONS:

- ➤ In a large sauté pan or skillet, heat the olive oil over medium heat
- ➤ Cook the onion for about 2 minutes, until fragrant
- ➤ Add the lamb and mix well, breaking up the meat as you cook
- ➤ Once the lamb is halfway cooked, add mint, parsley, red pepper flakes, and garlic powder.

- ➤ In a medium bowl, mix together the cooked rice and za'atar
- ➤ Then divide between individual serving bowls
- ➤ Join also the seasoned lamb
- ➤ Then top the bowls with the tomatoes, cucumber, hummus, feta, and pita (if using).

NUTRITION INFORMATION: Calories: 1312 fat: 96g protein: 62g carbs: 62g fiber: 12g sodium: 1454mg

19. BRAISED GARLIC FLANK STEAK WITH ARTICHOKES

Servings: 6   **Cook Time: 60 Min**   **Prep Time 15 Min**

INGREDIENTS:

- ✓ 4 tablespoons grapeseed oil, divided
- ✓ 2 pounds (907 g) flank steak
- ✓ 1 (14-ounce / 397-g) can artichoke hearts, drained and roughly chopped
- ✓ 1 onion, diced
- ✓ 8 garlic cloves, chopped
- ✓ 1 (32-ounce / 907-g) container low-sodium beef broth
- ✓ 1 (14½-ounce / 411-g) can diced tomatoes, drained
- ✓ 1 cup tomato sauce
- ✓ 2 tablespoons tomato paste
- ✓ 1 teaspoon dried oregano
- ✓ 1 teaspoon dried parsley
- ✓ 1 teaspoon dried basil
- ✓ ½ teaspoon ground cumin
- ✓ 3 bay leaves
- ✓ 2 to 3 cups cooked couscous (optional)

DIRECTIONS:

- ➤ Preheat the oven to 450°F (235°C).
- ➤ In an oven-safe sauté pan or skillet, heat 3 tablespoons of oil on medium heat
- ➤ Sear the steak for 2 minutes per side on both sides
- ➤ Transfer the steak to the oven for 30 minutes, or until desired tenderness.
- ➤ Meanwhile, in a large pot, combine the remaining 1 tablespoon of oil, artichoke hearts, onion, and garlic
- ➤ Pour in the beef broth, tomatoes, tomato sauce, and tomato paste
- ➤ Stir in oregano, parsley, basil, cumin, and bay leaves.
- ➤ Cook the vegetables, covered, for 30 minutes
- ➤ Remove bay leaf and serve with flank steak and ½ cup of couscous per plate, if using.

NUTRITION INFORMATION: Calories: 577 fat: 28g protein: 55g carbs: 22g fiber: 6g sodium: 1405mg

20. TRADITIONAL CHICKEN SHAWARMA

Servings: 6   **Cook Time: 15 Min**   **Prep Time 15 Min**

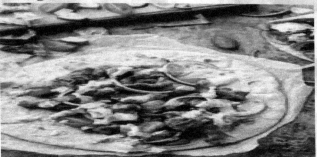

INGREDIENTS:

- ✓ 2 pounds (907 g) boneless and skinless chicken
- ✓ ½ cup lemon juice
- ✓ ½ cup extra-virgin olive oil
- ✓ 3 tablespoons minced garlic
- ✓ 1½ teaspoons salt
- ✓ ½ teaspoon freshly ground black pepper
- ✓ ½ teaspoon ground cardamom
- ✓ ½ teaspoon cinnamon
- ✓ Hummus and pita bread, for serving (optional)

DIRECTIONS:

- ➤ Cut the chicken into ¼-inch strips and put them into a large bowl.
- ➤ In a separate bowl, whisk together the lemon juice, olive oil
- ➤ Then garlic, salt, pepper, cardamom, and cinnamon.
- ➤ Pour the dressing over the chicken and stir to coat all of the chicken.
- ➤ Let the chicken sit for about 10 minutes.
- ➤ Heat a large pan over medium-high heat
- ➤ Cook the chicken pieces for 12 minutes, using tongs to turn the chicken over every few minutes.
- ➤ Serve with hummus and pita bread, if desired.

NUTRITION INFORMATION: Calories: 477 | fat: 32g | protein: 47g | carbs: 5g | fiber: 1g | sodium: 1234mg

21. CHICKEN SHISH TAWOOK

Servings: 6   **Cook Time: 15 Min**   **Prep Time 15 Min**

INGREDIENTS:

- ✓ 2 tablespoons garlic, minced
- ✓ 2 tablespoons tomato paste
- ✓ 1 teaspoon smoked paprika
- ✓ ½ cup lemon juice
- ✓ ½ cup extra-virgin olive oil

- ✓ 1½ teaspoons salt
- ✓ ½ teaspoon freshly ground black pepper
- ✓ 2 pounds (907 g) boneless and skinless chicken (breasts or thighs)
- ✓ Rice, tzatziki, or hummus, for serving (optional)

DIRECTIONS:

- ➢ In a large bowl, add the garlic, tomato paste, paprika,
- ➢ Then lemon juice, olive oil, salt, and pepper and whisk to combine.
- ➢ Cut the chicken into ½-inch cubes
- ➢ Put them into the bowl; toss to coat with the marinade
- ➢ Set aside for at least 10 minutes.
- ➢ To grill, preheat the grill on high

- ➢ Thread the chicken onto skewers
- ➢ Cook for 3 minutes per side, for a total of 9 minutes.
- ➢ To cook in a pan, preheat the pan on high heat
- ➢ Add the chicken, and cook for 9 minutes, turning over the chicken using tongs.
- ➢ Serve the chicken with rice, tzatziki, or hummus, if desired.

NUTRITION INFORMATION: Calories: 482 fat: 32g protein: 47g carbs: 6g fiber: 1g sodium: 1298mg

22. LEMON-GARLIC WHOLE CHICKEN AND POTATOES

Servings: 6   **Cook Time: 45 Min**   **Prep Time 10 Min**

INGREDIENTS:

- ✓ 1 cup garlic, minced
- ✓ 1½ cups lemon juice
- ✓ 1 cup plus
- ✓ 2 tablespoons extra-virgin olive oil, divided
- ✓ 1½ teaspoons salt, divided
- ✓ 1 teaspoon freshly ground black pepper
- ✓ 1 whole chicken, cut into
- ✓ 8 pieces
- ✓ 1 pound (454 g) fingerling or red potatoes

DIRECTIONS:

- ➢ Preheat the oven to 400°F (205°C).
- ➢ In a large bowl, whisk together the garlic, lemon juice, 1 cup of olive oil, 1 teaspoon of salt, and pepper.
- ➢ Put the chicken in a large baking dish and pour half of the lemon sauce over the chicken
- ➢ Cover the baking dish with foil, and cook for 20 minutes.
- ➢ Cut the potatoes in half, and toss to coat with 2 tablespoons olive oil and 1 teaspoon of salt
- ➢ Put them on a baking sheet and bake for 20 minutes in the same oven as the chicken.

- ➢ Take both the chicken and potatoes out of the oven
- ➢ Use a spatula, transfer the potatoes to the baking dish with the chicken
- ➢ Pour the remaining sauce over the potatoes and chicken
- ➢ Bake for another 25 minutes.
- ➢ Transfer the chicken and potatoes to a serving dish
- ➢ Spoon the garlic- lemon sauce from the pan on top.

NUTRITION INFORMATION: Calories: 959 fat: 78g protein: 33g carbs: 37g fiber: 4g sodium: 1005mg

23. LEMON CHICKEN THIGHS WITH VEGETABLES

Servings: 4　　　　**Cook Time: 45 Min**　　　　**Prep Time 15 Min**

INGREDIENTS:

- ✓ 6 tablespoons extra-virgin olive oil, divided
- ✓ 4 large garlic cloves, crushed
- ✓ 1 tablespoon dried basil
- ✓ 1 tablespoon dried parsley
- ✓ 1 tablespoon salt
- ✓ ½ tablespoon thyme
- ✓ 4 skin-on, bone-in chicken thighs

- ✓ 6 medium portobello mushrooms, quartered
- ✓ 1 large zucchini, sliced
- ✓ 1 large carrot, thinly sliced
- ✓ ⅛ cup pitted Kalamata olives
- ✓ 8 pieces sun-dried tomatoes (optional)
- ✓ ½ cup dry white wine
- ✓ 1 lemon, sliced

DIRECTIONS:

- ➢ In a small bowl, combine 4 tablespoons of olive oil, the garlic cloves, basil, parsley, salt, and thyme
- ➢ Store half of the marinade in a jar and, in a bowl
- ➢ Combine the remaining half to marinate the chicken thighs for about 30 minutes.
- ➢ Preheat the oven to 425°F (220°C).
- ➢ In a large skillet or oven-safe pan, heat the remaining 2 tablespoons of olive oil over medium-high heat
- ➢ Sear the chicken for 3 to 5 minutes on each side until golden brown, and set aside.

- ➢ In the same pan, sauté portobello mushrooms, zucchini, and carrot for about 5 minutes
- ➢ (Or until lightly browned)
- ➢ Add the chicken thighs, olives, and sun-dried tomatoes (if using)
- ➢ Pour the wine over the chicken thighs.
- ➢ Cover the pan and cook for about 10 minutes over medium-low heat.
- ➢ Uncover the pan and transfer it to the oven
- ➢ Cook for 15 more minutes, or until the chicken skin is crispy and the juices run clear
- ➢ Top with lemon slices.

NUTRITION INFORMATION: Calories: 544 fat: 41g protein: 28g carbs: 20g fiber: 11g sodium: 1848mg

24. YOGURT-MARINATED CHICKEN

Servings: 2　　　　**Cook Time: 30 Min**　　　　**Prep Time 15 Min**

INGREDIENTS:

- ✓ ½ cup plain Greek yogurt 3 garlic cloves, minced
- ✓ 2 tablespoons minced fresh oregano (or 1 tablespoon dried oregano)
- ✓ Zest of 1 lemon

- ✓ 1 tablespoon olive oil
- ✓ ½ teaspoon salt
- ✓ 2 (4-ounce / 113-g) boneless, skinless chicken breasts

DIRECTIONS:

- ➢ In a medium bowl, add the yogurt, garlic, oregano, lemon zest, olive oil, and salt and stir to combine
- ➢ If the yogurt is very thick, you may need to add a few tablespoons of water or a squeeze of lemon juice to thin it a bit.
- ➢ Add the chicken to the bowl
- ➢ Toss it in the marinade to coat it well

- ➢ Cover and refrigerate the chicken for at least 30 minutes or up to overnight.
- ➢ Preheat the oven to 350°F (180°C) and set the rack to the middle position.
- ➢ Place the chicken in a baking dish and roast for 30 minutes
- ➢ (Or until chicken reaches an internal temperature of 165°F (74°C))

NUTRITION INFORMATION: Calories: 255 fat: 13g protein: 29g carbs: 8g fiber: 2g sodium: 694mg

25. FETA STUFFED CHICKEN BREASTS

Servings: 4   **Cook Time: 20 Min**   **Prep Time 10 Min**

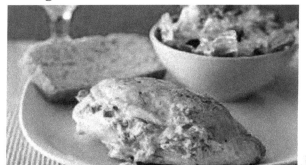

INGREDIENTS:

- ✓ ⅓ cup cooked brown rice
- ✓ 1 teaspoon shawarma seasoning
- ✓ 4 (6-ounce / 170-g) boneless skinless chicken breasts
- ✓ 1 tablespoon harissa
- ✓ 3 tablespoons extra-virgin olive oil, divided
- ✓ Salt and freshly ground black pepper, to taste
- ✓ 4 small dried apricots, halved
- ✓ ⅓ cup crumbled feta
- ✓ 1 tablespoon chopped fresh parsley

DIRECTIONS:

- ➤ Preheat the oven to 375°F (190°C).
- ➤ In a medium bowl, mix the rice and shawarma seasoning and set aside.
- ➤ Butterfly the chicken breasts by slicing them almost in half
- ➤ Start at the thickest part and folding them open like a book.
- ➤ In a small bowl, mix the harissa with 1 tablespoon of olive oil
- ➤ Brush the chicken with the harissa oil and season with salt and pepper
- ➤ The harissa adds a nice heat, so feel free to add a thicker coating for more spice.

- ➤ Onto one side of each chicken breast, spoon 1 to 2 tablespoons of rice
- ➤ Then layer 2 apricot halves in each breast
- ➤ Divide the feta between the chicken breasts and fold the other side over the filling to close.
- ➤ In an oven-safe sauté pan or skillet, heat the remaining 2 tablespoons of olive oil
- ➤ Sear the breast for 2 minutes on each side
- ➤ Then place the pan into the oven for 15 minutes, or until fully cooked and juices run clear
- ➤ Serve, garnished with parsley.

NUTRITION INFORMATION: Calories: 321 fat: 17g protein: 37g carbs: 8g fiber: 1g sodium: 410mg

26. CHICKEN SAUSAGE AND TOMATO WITH FARRO

Servings: 2   **Cook Time: 45 Min**   **Prep Time 10 Min**

INGREDIENTS:

- ✓ 1 tablespoon olive oil
- ✓ ½ medium onion, diced
- ✓ ¼ cup julienned sun-dried tomatoes packed in olive oil and herbs
- ✓ 8 ounces (227 g) hot Italian chicken sausage, removed from the casing

- ✓ ¾ cup farro
- ✓ 1½ cups low-sodium chicken stock
- ✓ 2 cups loosely packed arugula
- ✓ 4 to 5 large fresh basil leaves, sliced thin
- ✓ Salt, to taste

DIRECTIONS:

- ➤ Heat the olive oil in a sauté pan over medium-high heat
- ➤ Add the onion and sauté for 5 minutes
- ➤ Then the sun-dried tomatoes and chicken sausage
- ➤ Stir to break up the sausage
- ➤ Cook for 7 minutes, or until the sausage is no longer pink.
- ➤ Stir in the farro. Let it toast for 3 minutes, stirring occasionally.

- ➤ Join also the chicken stock and bring the mixture to a boil
- ➤ Cover the pan and reduce the heat to medium-low
- ➤ Let it simmer for 30 minutes, or until the farro is tender.
- ➤ Stir in the arugula and let it wilt slightly
- ➤ Add the basil, and season with salt.

NUTRITION INFORMATION: Calories: 491 fat: 18g protein: 31g carbs: 53g fiber: 6g sodium: 765mg

27. CHICKEN, MUSHROOMS, AND TARRAGON PASTA

Servings: 2   **Cook Time: 15 Min**   **Prep Time 15 Min**

INGREDIENTS:

- ✓ 2 tablespoons olive oil, divided
- ✓ ½ medium onion, minced
- ✓ 4 ounces (113 g) baby bella (cremini) mushrooms, sliced
- ✓ 2 small garlic cloves, minced
- ✓ 8 ounces (227 g) chicken cutlets
- ✓ 2 teaspoons tomato paste
- ✓ 2 teaspoons dried tarragon
- ✓ 2 cups low-sodium chicken stock 6 ounces (170 g) pappardelle pasta
- ✓ ¼ cup plain full-fat Greek yogurt
- ✓ Salt, to taste
- ✓ Freshly ground black pepper, to taste

DIRECTIONS:

- ➤ Heat 1 tablespoon of the olive oil in a sauté pan over medium-high heat
- ➤ Add the onion and mushrooms and sauté for 5 minutes
- ➤ Then the garlic and cook for 1 minute more.
- ➤ Move the vegetables to the edges of the pan
- ➤ Add the remaining 1 tablespoon of olive oil to the center of the pan
- ➤ Place the cutlets in the center and let them cook for about 3 minutes
- ➤ (Or until they lift up easily and are golden brown on the bottom)
- ➤ Flip the chicken and cook for another 3 minutes.
- ➤ Mix in the tomato paste and tarragon
- ➤ Then the chicken stock and stir well to combine everything
- ➤ Bring the stock to a boil.
- ➤ Add the pappardelle
- ➤ Break up the pasta if needed to fit into the pan
- ➤ Stir the noodles so they don't stick to the bottom of the pan.
- ➤ Cover the sauté pan and reduce the heat to medium-low
- ➤ Let the chicken and noodles simmer for 15 minutes, stirring occasionally
- ➤ (Until the pasta is cooked and the liquid is mostly absorbed)
- ➤ If the liquid absorbs too quickly and the pasta isn't cooked, add more water or chicken stock, about ¼ cup at a time as needed.
- ➤ Remove the pan from the heat.
- ➤ Stir 2 tablespoons of the hot liquid from the pan into the yogurt
- ➤ Pour the tempered yogurt into the pan
- ➤ Stir well to mix it into the sauce. Season with salt and pepper.
- ➤ The sauce will tighten up as it cools, so if it seems too thick, add a few tablespoons of water.

NUTRITION INFORMATION: Calories: 556 | fat: 17g | protein: 42g | carbs: 56g | fiber: 1g | sodium: 190mg

28. POACHED CHICKEN BREAST WITH ROMESCO SAUCE

Servings: 6 **Cook Time: 12 Min** **Prep Time 10 Min**

INGREDIENTS:

- ✓ 1½ pounds (680 g) boneless, skinless chicken breasts, cut into 6 pieces
- ✓ 1 carrot, halved
- ✓ 1 celery stalk, halved
- ✓ ½ onion, halved
- ✓ 2 garlic cloves, smashed
- ✓ 3 sprigs fresh thyme or rosemary
- ✓ 1 cup romesco sauce
- ✓ 2 tablespoons chopped fresh flat-leaf (Italian) parsley
- ✓ ¼ teaspoon freshly ground black pepper

DIRECTIONS:

- ➢ Put the chicken in a medium saucepan
- ➢ Fill with water until there's about one inch of liquid above the chicken
- ➢ Add the carrot, celery, onion, garlic, and thyme
- ➢ Cover and bring it to a boil
- ➢ Reduce the heat to low (keeping it covered), and cook for 12 to 15 minutes
- ➢ (Or until the internal temperature of the chicken measures 165°F (74°C) on a meat thermometer and any juices run clear)
- ➢ Remove the chicken from the water and let sit for 5 minutes.
- ➢ When you're ready to serve
- ➢ Spread ¾ cup of romesco sauce on the bottom of a serving platter
- ➢ Arrange the chicken breasts on top
- ➢ Drizzle with the remaining romesco sauce
- ➢ Sprinkle the tops with parsley and pepper.

NUTRITION INFORMATION: Calories: 270 fat: 10g protein: 13g carbs: 31g fiber: 2g sodium: 647mg

29. TAHINI CHICKEN RICE BOWLS WITH APRICOTS

Servings: 4 **Cook Time: 15 Min** **Prep Time 15 Min**

INGREDIENTS:

- ✓ 1 cup uncooked instant brown rice
- ✓ ¼ cup tahini or peanut butter (tahini for nut-free)
- ✓ ¼ cup 2% plain Greek yogurt
- ✓ 2 tablespoons chopped scallions, green and white parts
- ✓ 1 tablespoon freshly squeezed lemon juice
- ✓ 1 tablespoon water
- ✓ 1 teaspoon ground cumin
- ✓ ¾ teaspoon ground cinnamon
- ✓ ¼ teaspoon kosher or sea salt
- ✓ 2 cups chopped cooked chicken breast
- ✓ ½ cup chopped dried apricots
- ✓ 2 cups peeled and chopped seedless cucumber
- ✓ 4 teaspoons sesame seeds
- ✓ Fresh mint leaves, for serving (optional)

DIRECTIONS:

- ➢ Cook the brown rice according to the package instructions.
- ➢ While the rice is cooking, in a medium bowl
- ➢ Mix together the tahini, yogurt, scallions, lemon juice, water, cumin, cinnamon, and salt
- ➢ Transfer half the tahini mixture to another medium bowl
- ➢ Mix the chicken into the first bowl.
- ➢ When the rice is done, mix it into the second bowl of tahini
- ➢ (The one without the chicken).
- ➢ To assemble, divide the chicken among four bowls
- ➢ Spoon the rice mixture next to the chicken in each bowl
- ➢ Next to the chicken, place the dried apricots, and in the remaining empty section, add the cucumbers
- ➢ Sprinkle with sesame seeds, and top with mint, if desired, and serve.

NUTRITION INFORMATION: Calories: 335 fat: 10g protein: 31g carbs: 30g fiber: 3g sodium: 345mg

30. ROASTED ARTICHOKES WITH CHICKEN THIGH

Servings: 4   **Cook Time: 20 Min**   **Prep Time 5 Min**

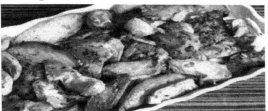

INGREDIENTS:

- ✓ 2 large lemons
- ✓ 3 tablespoons extra-virgin olive oil, divided
- ✓ ½ teaspoon kosher or sea salt
- ✓ 2 large artichokes
- ✓ 4 (6-ounce / 170-g) bone-in, skin-on chicken thighs

DIRECTIONS:

- ➢ Put a large, rimmed baking sheet in the oven
- ➢ Preheat the oven to 450°F (235°C) with the pan inside
- ➢ Tear off four sheets of aluminum foil about 8-by-10 inches each; set aside.
- ➢ Use a Microplane or citrus zester, zest 1 lemon into a large bowl
- ➢ Halve both lemons and squeeze all the juice into the bowl with the zest
- ➢ Whisk in 2 tablespoons of oil and the salt. Set aside.
- ➢ Rinse the artichokes with cool water, and dry with a clean towel
- ➢ Use a sharp knife, cut about 1½ inches off the tip of each artichoke
- ➢ Cut about ¼ inch off each stem
- ➢ Halve each artichoke lengthwise so each piece has equal amounts of stem
- ➢ Immediately plunge the artichoke halves into the lemon juice and oil mixture (To prevent browning)
- ➢ Turn to coat on all sides
- ➢ Lay one artichoke half flat-side down in the center of a sheet of aluminum foil
- ➢ Close up loosely to make a foil packet
- ➢ Repeat the process with the remaining three artichoke halves. Set the packets aside.
- ➢ Put the chicken in the remaining lemon juice mixture and turn to coat
- ➢ Use oven mitts, carefully remove the hot baking sheet from the oven
- ➢ Pour on the remaining tablespoon of oil; tilt the pan to coat
- ➢ Carefully arrange the chicken, skin-side down, on the hot baking sheet
- ➢ Place the artichoke packets, flat-side down, on the baking sheet as well
- ➢ (Arrange the artichoke packets and chicken with space between them so air can circulate around them.)
- ➢ Roast for 20 minutes
- ➢ (Or until the internal temperature of the chicken measures 165°F (74°C) on a meat thermometer and any juices run clear)
- ➢ Before serving, check the artichokes for doneness by pulling on a leaf
- ➢ If it comes out easily, the artichoke is ready.

NUTRITION INFORMATION: Calories: 832 | fat: 79g | protein: 19g | carbs: 11g | fiber: 4g | sodium: 544mg

31. CHICKEN BREAST WITH TOMATO AND BASIL

Servings: 4   **Cook Time: 20 Min**   **Prep Time 10**

INGREDIENTS:

- ✓ Nonstick cooking spray
- ✓ 1 pound (454 g) boneless, skinless chicken breasts
- ✓ 2 tablespoons extra-virgin olive oil
- ✓ ¼ teaspoon freshly ground black pepper
- ✓ ¼ teaspoon kosher or sea salt
- ✓ 1 large tomato, sliced thinly

- ✓ 1 cup shredded Mozzarella or 4 ounces fresh Mozzarella cheese, diced
- ✓ 1 (14½-ounce / 411-g) can low-sodium or no-salt-added crushed tomatoes
- ✓ 2 tablespoons fresh torn basil leaves
- ✓ 4 teaspoons balsamic vinegar

DIRECTIONS:

- ➢ Set one oven rack about 4 inches below the broiler element
- ➢ Preheat the oven to 450°F (235°C)
- ➢ Line a large, rimmed baking sheet with aluminum foil
- ➢ Place a wire cooling rack on the aluminum foil
- ➢ Spray the rack with nonstick cooking spray. Set aside.
- ➢ Cut the chicken into 4 pieces (if they aren't already)
- ➢ Put the chicken breasts in a large zip-top plastic bag
- ➢ With a rolling pin or meat mallet, pound the chicken so it is evenly flattened, about ¼-inch thick
- ➢ Add the oil, pepper, and salt to the bag
- ➢ Reseal the bag, and massage the ingredients into the chicken
- ➢ Take the chicken out of the bag and place it on the prepared wire rack.

- ➢ Cook the chicken for 15 to 18 minutes
- ➢ (Or until the internal temperature of the chicken is 165°F (74°C) on a meat thermometer and the juices run clear)
- ➢ Turn the oven to the high broiler setting
- ➢ Layer the tomato slices on each chicken breast, and top with the Mozzarella.
- ➢ Broil the chicken for another 2 to 3 minutes
- ➢ (Or until the cheese is melted)
- ➢ (Don't let the chicken burn on the edges)
- ➢ Remove the chicken from the oven
- ➢ While the chicken is cooking, pour the crushed tomatoes into a small, microwave-safe bowl
- ➢ Cover the bowl with a paper towel, and microwave for about 1 minute on high, until hot
- ➢ When you're ready to serve, divide the tomatoes among four dinner plates
- ➢ Place each chicken breast on top of the tomatoes
- ➢ Top with the basil and a drizzle of balsamic vinegar.

NUTRITION INFORMATION: Calories: 258 fat: 9g protein: 14g carbs: 28g fiber: 3g sodium: 573mg

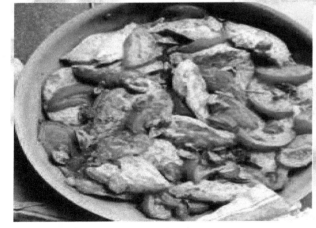

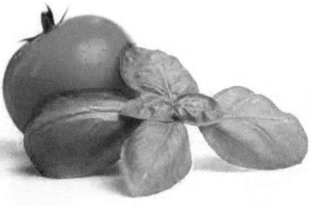

32. MASCARPONE WITH FIG CROSTINI

Servings: 8   **Cook Time: 10 Min**   **Prep Time 10 Min**

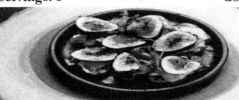

INGREDIENTS:
- ✓ 1 long French baguette
- ✓ 4 tablespoons (½ stick) salted butter, melted (optional)
- ✓ 1 (8-ounce / 227-g) tub mascarpone cheese
- ✓ 1 (12-ounce / 340-g) jar fig jam or preserves

DIRECTIONS:
- ➢ Preheat the oven to 350°F (180°C).
- ➢ Slice the bread into ¼-inch-thick slices.
- ➢ Arrange the sliced bread on a baking sheet and brush each slice with the melted butter (if desired).
- ➢ Put the baking sheet in the oven and toast the bread for 5 to 7 minutes, just until golden brown.
- ➢ Let the bread cool slightly
- ➢ Spread about a teaspoon or so of the mascarpone cheese on each piece of bread.
- ➢ Top with a teaspoon or so of the jam. Serve immediately.

NUTRITION INFORMATION: Calories: 445 fat: 24g protein: 3g carbs: 48g fiber: 5g sodium: 314mg

33. SESAME SEED COOKIES

Cookies: 16   **Cook Time: 15 Min**   **Prep Time 10 Min**

INGREDIENTS:
- ✓ 1 cup sesame seeds, hulled 1 cup sugar
- ✓ 8 tablespoons (1 stick) salted butter, softened (optional)
- ✓ 2 large eggs
- ✓ 1¼ cups flour

DIRECTIONS:
- ➢ Preheat the oven to 350°F (180°C)
- ➢ Toast the sesame seeds on a baking sheet for 3 minutes
- ➢ Set aside and let cool.
- ➢ Use a mixer, cream together the sugar and butter (if desired)
- ➢ Add the eggs one at a time until well-blended.
- ➢ Then the flour and toasted sesame seeds and mix until well-blended
- ➢ Drop spoonfuls of cookie dough onto a baking sheet
- ➢ Form them into round balls, about 1-inch in diameter, similar to a walnut.
- ➢ Put in the oven and bake for 5 to 7 minutes or until golden brown
- ➢ Let the cookies cool and enjoy.

NUTRITION INFORMATION: Calories: 218 fat: 12g protein: 4g carbs: 25g fiber: 2g sodium: 58mg

34. BUTTERY ALMOND COOKIES

Servings: 6   **Cook Time: 10 Min**   **Prep Time 5 Min**

INGREDIENTS:
- ✓ ½ cup sugar
- ✓ 8 tablespoons (1 stick) room temperature salted butter (optional)
- ✓ 1 large egg
- ✓ 1½ cups all-purpose flour
- ✓ cup ground almonds or almond flour

DIRECTIONS:
- ➢ Preheat the oven to 375°F (190°C).
- ➢ Use a mixer, cream together the sugar and butter (if desired).
- ➢ Add the egg and mix until combined.
- ➢ Alternately add the flour and ground almonds, ½ cup at a time, while the mixer is on slow.
- ➢ Once everything is combined, line a baking sheet with parchment paper
- ➢ Drop a tablespoon of dough on the baking sheet, keeping the cookies at least 2 inches apart.
- ➢ Put the baking sheet in the oven
- ➢ Bake just until the cookies start to turn brown around the edges, about 5 to 7 minutes

NUTRITION INFORMATION: Calories: 604 fat: 36g protein: 11g carbs: 63g fiber: 4g sodium: 181mg

35. HONEY WALNUT BAKLAVA

Servings: 8   **Cook Time: 1 H**   **Prep Time 30 Min**

INGREDIENTS:

- ✓ 2 cups very finely chopped walnuts or pecans
- ✓ 1 teaspoon cinnamon
- ✓ 1 cup (2 sticks) unsalted butter, melted (optional)
- ✓ 1 (16-ounce / 454-g) package phyllo dough, thawed
- ✓ 1 (12-ounce / 340-g) jar honey

DIRECTIONS:

- ➢ Preheat the oven to 350°F (180°C).
- ➢ In a bowl, combine the chopped nuts and cinnamon.
- ➢ Use a brush, butter the sides and bottom of a 9-by-13-inch inch baking dish.
- ➢ Remove the phyllo dough from the package
- ➢ Cut it to the size of the baking dish using a sharp knife.
- ➢ Place one sheet of phyllo dough on the bottom of the dish
- ➢ Brush with butter, and repeat until you have 8 layers.
- ➢ Sprinkle ⅓ cup of the nut mixture over the phyllo layers
- ➢ Top with a sheet of phyllo dough, butter that sheet
- ➢ Repeat until you have 4 sheets of buttered phyllo dough.
- ➢ Sprinkle ⅓ cup of the nut mixture for another layer of nuts
- ➢ Repeat the layering of nuts and 4 sheets of buttered phyllo until all the nut mixture is gone
- ➢ The last layer should be 8 buttered sheets of phyllo.
- ➢ Before you bake, cut the baklava into desired shapes; traditionally this is diamonds, triangles, or squares.
- ➢ Bake the baklava for 1 hour or until the top layer is golden brown.
- ➢ While the baklava is baking, heat the honey in a pan just until it is warm and easy to pour.
- ➢ Once the baklava is done baking, immediately
- ➢ Pour the honey evenly over the baklava and let it absorb it, about 20 minutes
- ➢ Serve warm or at room temperature

NUTRITION INFORMATION: Calories: 754 fat: 46g protein: 8g carbs: 77g fiber: 3g sodium: 33mg

36. CREAMY RICE PUDDING

Servings: 6   **Cook Time: 45 Min**   **Prep Time 5 Min**

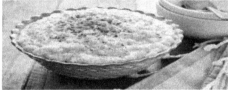

INGREDIENTS:

- ✓ 1¼ cups long-grain rice
- ✓ 5 cups unsweetened almond milk
- ✓ 1 cup sugar
- ✓ 1 tablespoon rose water or orange blossom water
- ✓ 1 teaspoon cinnamon

DIRECTIONS:

- ➢ Rinse the rice under cold water for 30 seconds.
- ➢ Put the rice, milk, and sugar in a large pot
- ➢ Bring to a gentle boil while continually stirring.
- ➢ Turn the heat down to low and let simmer for 40 to 45 minutes
- ➢ Stir every 3 to 4 minutes so that the rice does not stick to the bottom of the pot.
- ➢ Add the rose water at the end and simmer for 5 minutes.
- ➢ Divide the pudding into 6 bowls
- ➢ Sprinkle the top with cinnamon
- ➢ Cool for at least 1 hour before serving. Store in the fridge.

NUTRITION INFORMATION: Calories: 323 fat: 7g protein: 9g carbs: 56g fiber: 1g sodium: 102mg

37. CREAM CHEESE AND RICOTTA CHEESECAKE

Servings: 10 **Cook Time: 1 H** **Prep Time 5 Min**

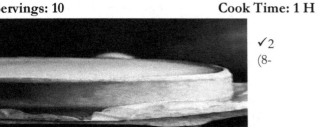

✓ 2 (8- ounce / 227-g) packages full-fat cream cheese

INGREDIENTS:

- ✓ 1 (16-ounce / 454-g) container full-fat ricotta cheese
- ✓ 1½ cups granulated sugar
- ✓ 1 tablespoon lemon zest
- ✓ 5 large eggs
- ✓ Nonstick cooking spray

DIRECTIONS:

- ➤ Preheat the oven to 350ºF (180ºC).
- ➤ Use a mixer, blend together the cream cheese and ricotta cheese.
- ➤ Blend in the sugar and lemon zest.
- ➤ Blend in the eggs; drop in 1 egg at a time, blend for 10 seconds, and repeat.
- ➤ Line a 9-inch springform pan with parchment paper and nonstick spray
- ➤ Wrap the bottom of the pan with foil
- ➤ Pour the cheesecake batter into the pan.
- ➤ To make a water bath, get a baking or roasting pan larger than the cheesecake pan
- ➤ Fill the roasting pan about ⅓ of the way up with warm water
- ➤ Put the cheesecake pan into the water bath
- ➤ Place the whole thing in the oven
- ➤ Let the cheesecake bake for 1 hour.
- ➤ After baking is complete, remove the cheesecake pan from the water bath and remove the foil
- ➤ Let the cheesecake cool for 1 hour on the countertop
- ➤ Then put it in the fridge to cool for at least 3 hours before serving.

NUTRITION INFORMATION: Calories: 489 fat: 31g protein: 15g carbs: 42g fiber: 0g sodium: 264mg

38. VANILLA CAKE BITES

Makes 24 bites **Cook Time: 45 Min** **Prep Time 10 Min**

INGREDIENTS:

- ✓ 1 (12-ounce / 340-g) box butter cake mix
- ✓ ½ cup (1 stick) butter, melted (optional)
- ✓ 3 large eggs, divided
- ✓ 1 cup sugar
- ✓ 1 (8-ounce / 227-g) cream cheese
- ✓ 1 teaspoon vanilla extract

DIRECTIONS:

- ➤ Preheat the oven to 350ºF (180ºC).
- ➤ To make the first layer, in a medium bowl
- ➤ Blend the cake mix, butter (if desired), and 1 egg
- ➤ Then, pour the mixture into the prepared pan.
- ➤ In a separate bowl, to make layer 2, mix together sugar, cream cheese
- ➤ Add the remaining 2 eggs, and vanilla
- ➤ Pour this gently over the first layer
- ➤ Bake for 45 to 50 minutes and allow to cool.
- ➤ Cut the cake into 24 small squares.

NUTRITION INFORMATION: Calories: 160 fat: 8g protein: 2g carbs: 20g fiber: 0g sodium: 156mg

39. CRANBERRY ORANGE LOAF

Makes 1 loaf   **Cook Time: 45 Min**   **Prep Time 20 Min**

INGREDIENTS:

DOUGH:

- ✓ 3 cups all-purpose flour
- ✓ 1 (¼-ounce / 7-g) package quick-rise yeast
- ✓ ½ teaspoon salt
- ✓ ⅛ teaspoon ground cinnamon
- ✓ ⅛ teaspoon ground cardamom

- ✓ ½ cup water
- ✓ ½ cup almond milk
- ✓ ⅓ cup butter, cubed (optional)

CRANBERRY FILLING:

- ✓ 1 (12-ounce / 340-g) can cranberry sauce
- ✓ ½ cup chopped walnuts

- ✓ 2 tablespoons grated orange zest
- ✓ 2 tablespoons orange juice

DIRECTIONS:

- ➤ In a large bowl, combine the flour, yeast, salt, cinnamon, and cardamom.
- ➤ In a small pot, heat the water, almond milk, and butter (if desired) over medium-high heat
- ➤ Once it boils, reduce the heat to medium-low
- ➤ Simmer for 10 to 15 minutes, until the liquid thickens.

- ➤ Pour the liquid ingredients into the dry ingredients
- ➤ Use a wooden spoon or spatula
- ➤ Mix the dough until it forms a ball in the bowl.
- ➤ Put the dough in a greased bowl
- ➤ Cover tightly with a kitchen towel, and set aside for 1 hour.

TO MAKE THE CRANBERRY FILLING:

- ➤ In a medium bowl, mix the cranberry sauce with walnuts
- ➤ Add orange zest, and orange juice in a large bowl.
- ➤ Assemble the bread
- ➤ Roll out the dough to about a 1-inch-thick and 10-by-7-inch-wide rectangle.
- ➤ Spread the cranberry filling evenly on the surface of the rolled-out dough
- ➤ Leave a 1-inch border around the edges

- ➤ Starting with the long side, tuck the dough under with your fingertips and roll up the dough tightly
- ➤ Place the rolled-up dough in an "S" shape in a bread pan.
- ➤ Allow the bread to rise again, about 30 to 40 minutes.
- ➤ Preheat the oven to 350°F (180°C).
- ➤ Bake in a preheated oven, 45 minutes.

NUTRITION INFORMATION: Calories: 483 fat: 15g protein: 8g carbs: 79g fiber: 4g sodium: 232mg

40. APPLE PIE POCKETS

Servings: 6   **Cook Time: 15 Min**   **Prep Time 5 Min**

INGREDIENTS:

- ✓ 1 organic puff pastry, rolled out, at room temperature
- ✓ 1 Gala apple, peeled and sliced
- ✓ ¼ cup brown sugar

- ✓ ⅛ teaspoon ground cinnamon
- ✓ ⅛ teaspoon ground cardamom
- ✓ Nonstick cooking spray
- ✓ Honey, for topping

DIRECTIONS:

- ➤ Preheat the oven to 350°F (180°C).
- ➤ Cut the pastry dough into 4 even discs
- ➤ Peel and slice the apple
- ➤ In a small bowl, toss the slices with brown sugar, cinnamon, and cardamom.
- ➤ Spray a muffin tin very well with nonstick cooking spray

- ➤ Be sure to spray only the muffin holders you plan to use.
- ➤ Once sprayed, line the bottom of the muffin tin with the dough
- ➤ Place 1 or 2 broken apple slices on top
- ➤ Fold the remaining dough over the apple and drizzle with honey.
- ➤ Bake for 15 minutes or until brown and bubbly.

NUTRITION INFORMATION: Calories: 250 fat: 15g protein: 3g carbs: 30g fiber: 1g sodium: 98mg

41. BAKED PEARS WITH MASCARPONE CHEESE

Servings: 2 **Cook Time: 20 Min** **Prep Time 10 Min**

INGREDIENTS:

- ✓ 2 ripe pears, peeled
- ✓ 1 tablespoon plus 2 teaspoons honey, divided
- ✓ 1 teaspoon vanilla, divided
- ✓ ¼ teaspoon ginger
- ✓ ¼ teaspoon ground coriander
- ✓ ¼ cup minced walnuts
- ✓ ¼ cup mascarpone cheese
- ✓ Pinch salt

DIRECTIONS:

- ➤ Preheat the oven to 350°F (180°C)
- ➤ Set the rack to the middle position. Grease a small baking dish.
- ➤ Cut the pears in half lengthwise
- ➤ Use a spoon, scoop out the core from each piece
- ➤ Place the pears with the cut side up in the baking dish.
- ➤ Combine 1 tablespoon of honey, ½ teaspoon of vanilla
- ➤ Add ginger, and coriander in a small bowl
- ➤ Pour this mixture evenly over the pear halves.
- ➤ Sprinkle walnuts over the pear halves.
- ➤ Bake for 20 minutes, or until the pears are golden and you're able to pierce them easily with a knife.
- ➤ While the pears are baking, mix the mascarpone cheese with the remaining 2 teaspoons honey, ½ teaspoon of vanilla, and a pinch of salt
- ➤ Stir well to combine.
- ➤ Divide the mascarpone among the warm pear halves and serve.

NUTRITION INFORMATION: Calories: 307 fat: 16g protein: 4g carbs: 43g fiber: 6g sodium: 89mg

42. ORANGE MUG CAKE

Servings: 2 **Cook Time: 2 Min** **Prep Time 10 Min**

INGREDIENTS:

- ✓ 6 tablespoons flour
- ✓ 2 tablespoons sugar
- ✓ ½ teaspoon baking powder
- ✓ Pinch salt
- ✓ 1 teaspoon orange zest
- ✓ 1 egg
- ✓ 2 tablespoons olive oil
- ✓ 2 tablespoons freshly squeezed orange juice
- ✓ 2 tablespoons unsweetened almond milk
- ✓ ½ teaspoon orange extract
- ✓ ½ teaspoon vanilla extract

DIRECTIONS:

- ➤ In a small bowl, combine the flour, sugar, baking powder, salt, and orange zest.
- ➤ In a separate bowl, whisk together the egg, olive oil, orange juice, milk, orange extract, and vanilla extract.
- ➤ Pour the dry ingredients into the wet ingredients
- ➤ Stir to combine. The batter will be thick.
- ➤ Divide the mixture into two small mugs that hold at least 6 ounces / 170 g each, or 1 (12-ounce / 340-g) mug.
- ➤ Microwave each mug separately
- ➤ The small ones should take about 60 seconds, and one large mug should take about 90 seconds, but microwaves can vary
- ➤ The cake will be done when it pulls away from the sides of the mug.

NUTRITION INFORMATION: Calories: 302 fat: 17g protein: 6g carbs: 33g fiber: 1g sodium: 117mg

43. FRUIT AND NUT DARK CHOCOLATE BARK

Servings: 2　　　　　　　**Cook Time: 5 Min**　　　　　　**Prep Time 15 Min**

INGREDIENTS:

- ✓ 2 tablespoons chopped nuts (almonds, pecans, walnuts, hazelnuts, pistachios, or any combination of those)
- ✓ 3 ounces (85 g) good-quality dark chocolate chips (about ⅔ cup)
- ✓ ¼ cup chopped dried fruit (apricots, blueberries, figs, prunes, or any combination of those)

DIRECTIONS:

- ➢ Line a sheet pan with parchment paper.
- ➢ Place the nuts in a skillet over medium-high
- ➢ Heat and toast them for 60 seconds, or just until they're fragrant.
- ➢ Place the chocolate in a microwave-safe glass bowl or measuring cup and microwave on high for 1 minute
- ➢ Stir the chocolate and allow any unmelted chips to warm and melt
- ➢ If necessary, heat for another 20 to 30 seconds, but keep a close eye on it to make sure it doesn't burn.
- ➢ Pour the chocolate onto the sheet pan
- ➢ Sprinkle the dried fruit and nuts over the chocolate evenly and gently pat in so they stick.
- ➢ Transfer the sheet pan to the refrigerator for at least 1 hour to let the chocolate harden.
- ➢ When solid, break into pieces
- ➢ Store any leftover chocolate in the refrigerator or freezer.

NUTRITION INFORMATION: Calories: 284 fat: 16g protein: 4g carbs: 39g fiber: 2g sodium: 2mg

44. GRILLED FRUIT SKEWERS

Servings: 2　　　　　　　**Cook Time: 10 Min**　　　　　　**Prep Time 15 Min**

INGREDIENTS:

- ✓ ⅔ cup prepared labneh, or, if making your own, ⅔ cup full-fat plain Greek yogurt
- ✓ 2 tablespoons honey
- ✓ 1 teaspoon vanilla extract Pinch salt
- ✓ 3 cups fresh fruit cut into 2-inch chunks (pineapple, cantaloupe, nectarines, strawberries, plums, or mango)

DIRECTIONS:

- ➢ If making your own labneh, place a colander over a bowl and line it with cheesecloth
- ➢ Place the Greek yogurt in the cheesecloth and wrap it up
- ➢ Put the bowl in the refrigerator and let sit for at least 12 to 24 hours
- ➢ (Until it's thick like soft cheese)
- ➢ Mix honey, vanilla, and salt into labneh
- ➢ Stir well to combine and set it aside.
- ➢ Heat the grill to medium (about 300°F / 150°C) and oil the grill grate
- ➢ Alternatively, you can cook these on the stovetop in a heavy grill pan
- ➢ (cast iron works well).
- ➢ Thread the fruit onto skewers and grill for 4 minutes on each side
- ➢ (Or until fruit is softened and has grill marks on each side)
- ➢ Serve the fruit with labneh to dip.

NUTRITION INFORMATION: Calories: 292 fat: 6g protein: 5g carbs: 60g fiber: 4g sodium: 131mg

45. POMEGRANATE BLUEBERRY GRANITA

Servings: 2   **Cook Time: 10 Min**   **Prep Time 15 Min**

INGREDIENTS:

- ✓ 1 cup frozen wild blueberries
- ✓ 1 cup pomegranate or pomegranate blueberry juice
- ✓ ¼ cup sugar
- ✓ ¼ cup water

DIRECTIONS:

- ➤ Combine the frozen blueberries and pomegranate juice in a saucepan and bring to a boil
- ➤ Reduce the heat and simmer for 5 minutes
- ➤ (Or until the blueberries start to break down)
- ➤ While the juice and berries are cooking
- ➤ Combine the sugar and water in a small microwave-safe bowl
- ➤ Microwave for 60 seconds, or until it comes to a rolling boil
- ➤ Stir to make sure all of the sugar is dissolved and set the syrup aside
- ➤ Combine the blueberry mixture and the sugar syrup in a blender
- ➤ Blend for 1 minute, or until the fruit is completely puréed.
- ➤ Pour the mixture into an 8-by-8-inch baking pan or a similar-sized bowl
- ➤ The liquid should come about ½ inch up the sides
- ➤ Let the mixture cool for 30 minutes, and then put it into the freezer.
- ➤ Every 30 minutes for the next 2 hours
- ➤ Scrape the granita with a fork to keep it from freezing solid.
- ➤ Serve it after 2 hours, or store it in a covered container in the freezer.

NUTRITION INFORMATION: Calories: 214 fat: 0g protein: 1g carbs: 54g fiber: 2g sodium: 15mg

46. CHOCOLATE DESSERT HUMMUS

Servings: 2   **Cook Time: 0 Min**   **Prep Time 15 Min**

INGREDIENTS:

CARAMEL:

- ✓ 2 tablespoons coconut oil
- ✓ 1 tablespoon maple syrup

HUMMUS:

- ✓ ½ cup chickpeas, drained and rinsed
- ✓ 2 tablespoons unsweetened cocoa powder
- ✓ 1 tablespoon maple syrup, plus more to taste
- ✓ 1 tablespoon almond butter Pinch salt
- ✓ 2 tablespoons almond milk, or more as needed, to thin Pinch salt
- ✓ 2 tablespoons pecans

DIRECTIONS:

MAKE THE CARAMEL

- ➤ To make the caramel, put the coconut oil in a small microwave-safe bowl
- ➤ If it's solid, microwave it for about 15 seconds to melt it.

MAKE THE HUMMUS

- ➤ In a food processor, combine the chickpeas, cocoa powder
- ➤ Then maple syrup, almond milk, and pinch of salt, and process until smooth
- ➤ Scrape down the sides to make sure everything is incorporated.
- ➤ If the hummus seems too thick, add another tablespoon of almond milk.
- ➤ Stir in the maple syrup, almond butter, and salt.
- ➤ Place the caramel in the refrigerator for 5 to 10 minutes to thicken.

- ➤ Add the pecans and pulse 6 times to roughly chop them.
- ➤ Transfer the hummus to a serving bowl
- ➤ When the caramel is thickened, swirl it into the hummus
- ➤ Gently fold it in, but don't mix it in completely.
- ➤ Serve with fresh fruit or pretzels.

NUTRITION INFORMATION: Calories: 321 fat: 22g protein: 7g carbs: 30g fiber: 6g sodium: 100mg

47. BLACKBERRY LEMON PANNA COTTA

Servings: 2   **Cook Time: 10 Min**   **Prep Time 20 Min**

INGREDIENTS:

- ✓ ¾ cup half-and-half, divided
- ✓ 1 teaspoon unflavored powdered gelatin
- ✓ ½ cup heavy cream
- ✓ 3 tablespoons sugar
- ✓ 1 teaspoon lemon zest
- ✓ 1 tablespoon freshly squeezed lemon juice
- ✓ 1 teaspoon lemon extract
- ✓ ½ cup fresh blackberries
- ✓ Lemon peels to garnish (optional)

DIRECTIONS:

- ➢ Place ¼ cup of half-and-half in a small bowl.
- ➢ Sprinkle the gelatin powder evenly over the half-and-half and set it aside for 10 minutes to hydrate.
- ➢ In a saucepan, combine the remaining ½ cup of half-
- ➢ Add-half, the heavy cream, sugar, lemon zest, lemon juice, and lemon extract
- ➢ Heat the mixture over medium heat for 4 minutes, or until it's barely simmering
- ➢ (Don't let it come to a full boil)
- ➢ Remove from the heat.

- ➢ When the gelatin is hydrated (it will look like applesauce)
- ➢ Add it into the warm cream mixture, whisking as the gelatin melts.
- ➢ If there are any remaining clumps of gelatin
- ➢ Strain the liquid or remove the lumps with a spoon.
- ➢ Pour the mixture into 2 dessert glasses or stemless wineglasses
- ➢ Refrigerate for at least 6 hours, or up to overnight.
- ➢ Serve with the fresh berries and garnish with some strips of fresh lemon peel, if desired.

NUTRITION INFORMATION: Calories: 422 fat: 33g protein: 6g carbs: 28g fiber: 2g sodium: 64mg

48. BERRY AND HONEY COMPOTE

Servings: 3   **Cook Time: 5 Min**   **Prep Time 5 Min**

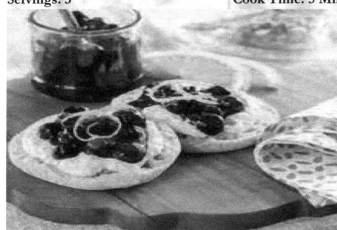

INGREDIENTS:
- ✓ ½ cup honey
- ✓ ¼ cup fresh berries
- ✓ 2 tablespoons grated orange zest

DIRECTIONS:
- ✓ 1.In a small saucepan, heat the honey, berries, and orange zest over medium-low heat for 2 to 5 minutes
- ✓ (Until the sauce thickens, or heat for 15 seconds in the microwave)
- ✓ Serve the compote drizzled over pancakes, muffins, or French toast.

NUTRITION INFORMATION: Calories: 272 fat: 0g protein: 1g carbs: 74g fiber: 1g sodium: 4mg

49. POMEGRANATE AND QUINOA DARK CHOCOLATE BARK

Servings: 6   **Cook Time: 13 Min**   **Prep Time 5 Min**

INGREDIENTS:

- ✓ Nonstick cooking spray
- ✓ ½ cup uncooked tricolor or regular quinoa
- ✓ ½ teaspoon kosher or sea salt
- ✓ 8 ounces (227 g) dark chocolate or 1 cup dark chocolate chips
- ✓ ½ cup fresh pomegranate seeds

DIRECTIONS:

- ➤ In a medium saucepan coated with nonstick cooking spray over medium heat
- ➤ Toast the uncooked quinoa for 2 to 3 minutes, stirring frequently
- ➤ Do not let the quinoa burn
- ➤ Remove the pan from the stove, and mix in the salt
- ➤ Set aside 2 tablespoons of the toasted quinoa to use for the topping.
- ➤ Break the chocolate into large pieces
- ➤ Put it in a gallon-size zip-top plastic bag
- ➤ Use a metal ladle or a meat pounder
- ➤ Pound the chocolate until broken into smaller pieces
- ➤ (If using chocolate chips, you can skip this step.)
- ➤ Dump the chocolate out of the bag into a medium, microwave
- ➤ (Safe bowl and heat for 1 minute on high in the microwave)
- ➤ Stir until the chocolate is completely melted
- ➤ Mix the toasted quinoa (except the topping you set aside) into the melted chocolate.
- ➤ Line a large, rimmed baking sheet with parchment paper
- ➤ Pour the chocolate mixture onto the sheet and spread it evenly
- ➤ (Until the entire pan is covered)
- ➤ Sprinkle the remaining 2 tablespoons of quinoa and the pomegranate seeds on top
- ➤ Use a spatula or the back of a spoon
- ➤ Press the quinoa and the pomegranate seeds into the chocolate.
- ➤ Freeze the mixture for 10 to 15 minutes, or until set
- ➤ Remove the bark from the freezer
- ➤ Break it into about 2-inch jagged pieces
- ➤ Store in a sealed container or zip-top plastic bag in the refrigerator until ready to serve.

NUTRITION INFORMATION: Calories: 268 fat: 11g protein: 4g carbs: 37g fiber: 2g sodium: 360mg

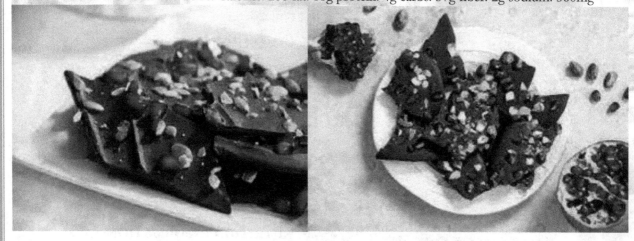

50. PECAN AND CARROT COCONUT CAKE

Servings: 12 **Cook Time: 45 Min** **Prep Time 10 Min**

INGREDIENTS:

- ✓ ½ cup coconut oil, at room temperature, plus more for greasing the baking dish
- ✓ 2 teaspoons pure vanilla extract
- ✓ ¼ cup pure maple syrup 6 eggs
- ✓ ½ cup coconut flour
- ✓ 1 teaspoon baking powder 1 teaspoon baking soda
- ✓ ½ teaspoon ground nutmeg 1 teaspoon ground cinnamon
- ✓ ⅛ teaspoon sea salt
- ✓ ½ cup chopped pecans
- ✓ 3 cups finely grated carrots

DIRECTIONS:

- ➢ Preheat the oven to 350°F (180°C). Grease a 13-by-9-inch baking dish with coconut oil.
- ➢ Combine the vanilla extract, maple syrup, and ½ cup of coconut oil in a large bowl. Stir to mix well.
- ➢ Break the eggs in the bowl and whisk to combine well. Set aside.
- ➢ Combine the coconut flour, baking powder, baking soda, nutmeg, cinnamon, and salt in a separate bowl
- ➢ Stir to mix well.
- ➢ Make a well in the center of the flour mixture
- ➢ Then pour the egg mixture into the well
- ➢ Stir to combine well.
- ➢ Add the pecans and carrots to the bowl and toss to mix wel
- ➢ Pour the mixture in the single layer on the baking dish.
- ➢ Bake in the preheated oven for 45 minutes or until puffed and the cake spring back when lightly press with your fingers.
- ➢ Remove the cake from the oven
- ➢ Allow to cool for at least 15 minutes, then serve.

NUTRITION INFORMATION: Calories: 255 fat: 21g protein: 5g carbs: 12g fiber: 2g sodium: 202mg

51. AVOCADOS CHOCOLATE PUDDING

Servings: 4 **Cook Time: 0 Min** **Prep Time 10 Min**

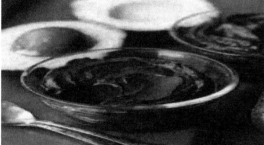

INGREDIENTS:

- ✓ 1 ripe avocados, halved and pitted
- ✓ ¼ cup unsweetened cocoa powder
- ✓ ¼ cup heavy whipping cream, plus more if needed
- ✓ 2 teaspoons vanilla extract
- ✓ 1 to 2 teaspoons liquid stevia or monk fruit extract (optional)
- ✓ ½ teaspoon ground cinnamon (optional)
- ✓ ¼ teaspoon salt
- ✓ Whipped cream, for serving (optional)

DIRECTIONS:

- ➢ Use a spoon, scoop out the ripe avocado into a blender or large bowl
- ➢ (If using an immersion blender)
- ➢ Mash well with a fork.
- ➢ Add the cocoa powder, heavy whipping cream, vanilla, sweetener (if using), cinnamon (if using), and salt
- ➢ Blend well until smooth and creamy, adding additional cream, 1 tablespoon at a time, if the mixture is too thick.
- ➢ Cover and refrigerate for at least 1 hour before serving
- ➢ Serve chilled with additional whipped cream, if desired

NUTRITION INFORMATION: Calories: 230 fat: 21g protein: 3g carbs: 10g fiber: 5g sodium: 163mg

52. GINGER CHICKEN TOASTED SESAME GINGER CHICKEN

Servings: 4   **Cook Time: 15Min**   **Prep Time 10 Min**

INGREDIENTS:

- ✓ 1 Tablespoon
- ✓ Toasted Sesame
- ✓ Ginger Seasoning (or toasted sesame seeds
- ✓ Garlic, onion powder
- ✓ Red pepper
- ✓ Ground ginger
- ✓ Salt
- ✓ Pepper
- ✓ Llemon
- ✓ 1 1/2 lbs. boneless, skinless chicken breast
- ✓ 4 teaspoons Olive Oil

DIRECTIONS:

- ➤ On a clean, dry cutting board put the chicken breasts.
- ➤ Softly flatten the chicken breasts to the approx. thickness of 3/8
- ➤ (Use a beef hammer or a frying pans backside)
- ➤ Dust with some seasoning.
- ➤ Heat the Olive Oil over medium-high flame in a big, nonstick frying pan.
- ➤ Add the chicken and cook on one side for about 7-8 minutes
- ➤ (Uuntil a beautiful crust has created ,it will be mildly orange)
- ➤ Turn the chicken softly and cook on the other side for a further 5-6 minutes
- ➤ (Before the chicken is thoroughly cooked)
- ➤ Serve hot or cooled over salad with your favorite side dish
- ➤ Makes about 4 servings.

NUTRITION INFORMATION: 310 kcal Protein: 16.14 g Fat: 10.64 g Carbohydrates: 36.65 g

53. TASTY AND TENDER FISH TACOS

Servings: 4   **Cook Time: 15Min**   **Prep Time 15 Min**

INGREDIENTS:

- ✓ 2 teaspoons Olive Oil (or oil)
- ✓ Fresh garlic
- ✓ 1 capful (1 Tablespoon)
- ✓ Southwestern Seasoning or Phoenix Sunrise
- ✓ Cumin
- ✓ Garlic
- ✓ Cilantro
- ✓ Red pepper
- ✓ Onion
- ✓ Parsley
- ✓ Paprika
- ✓ Salt & pepper (or low sodium taco seasoning)
- ✓ 1 3/4 lbs. cod or haddock (wild-caught)

DIRECTIONS:

- ➤ Clean your fish and slice into 1" pieces.
- ➤ Sprinkle with the seasoning
- ➤ Toss over to coat the fish thoroughly.
- ➤ Heat the Olive Oil over medium-high flame in a big, nonstickfrying pan.
- ➤ Add the fish and cook for about 10 to 12 minutes until the fish is transparent
- ➤ Splits into pieces. Be cautious not to overcook; otherwise, the fish may be dry and chewy.
- ➤ With your favorite condiments, serve warm.
- ➤ Makes about 4 servings.

NUTRITION INFORMATION: 748 kcal-Protein: 29.23 g-Fat: 6.64 g Carbohydrates 148.64 g

54. STUFFED SAUSAGE MUSHROOMS

Servings: 4   **Cook Time: 25Min**   **Prep Time 10 Min**

INGREDIENTS:

- ✓ 4 large Portobello mushrooms (caps and stems)
- ✓ 1 capful (1 Tablespoon)
- ✓ Garlic & Spring Onion Seasoning or Garlic Gusto Seasoning or chopped garlic
- ✓ Chopped chives, garlic powder
- ✓ Onion powder
- ✓ Salt, and pepper to taste
- ✓ 1 1/2 pounds lean Italian sausage (85-94% lean)

DIRECTIONS:

- ➢ Preheat the oven to 350 ° C
- ➢ Cut the mushroom stems carefully and clean both the tops and stems,
- ➢ The stems are chopped into tiny pieces
- ➢ Placed in a bowl Put the meat and spices to the bowl
- ➢ Mix all the spices well, using your fingertips
- ➢ Set the smooth side of the mushroom caps on a wide cookie sheet or baking tray.
- ➢ Divide 4 equal sections of the meat mixture
- ➢ Lightly press one section into each mushroom head.
- ➢ Bake with your favorite side dishes for about 25 minutes & serve crispy

NUTRITION INFORMATION: 437 kcal-Protein: 31.52 g-Fat: 30.89 g -Carbohydrates:16.74 g

55. SMOKY SHRIMP CHIPOTLE

Servings: 4   **Cook Time: 15Min**   **Prep Time 15 Min**

INGREDIENTS:

- ✓ 1 capful (1 Tablespoon)
- ✓ Cinnamon
- ✓ Chipotle or a small amount of chipotle pepper
- ✓ Cinnamon, salt, and pepper to taste
- ✓ Teaspoons Olive Oil
- ✓ Fresh garlic
- ✓ 4 T fresh cilantro (optional)
- ✓ 2 lbs. wild-caught
- ✓ Raw shrimp shelled
- ✓ Deveined & tails removed
- ✓ 1 can (16 oz.) diced tomatoes (unflavored, no sugar added)
- ✓ 1 C chopped chives or scallions (greens only)
- ✓ 4 lime wedges (optional)

DIRECTIONS:

- ➢ Heat oil over medium-high heat in a medium-sized frying pan.
- ➢ Put the scallions and roast, until mildly wilted and glistening,
- ➢ for one minute.
- ➢ Include the shrimp and cook on each side for 1 minute.
- ➢ Add the sauce with the tomatoes and Cinnamon Chipotle
- ➢ Cook an extra 3-5 minutes, stirring regularly
- ➢ (Until the tomatoes are hot and the shrimp is thoroughly cooked and opaque)
- ➢ Be careful not to overcook the shrimp which could become hard and dry
- ➢ If needed, sprinkle with cilantro and spritz with a wedge of lime
- ➢ (or for a beautiful and practical garnish
- ➢ Serve the lime wedge on the plate.
- ➢ Serve it warm.

NUTRITION INFORMATION: 632 kcal--Protein: 44.58 g--Fat: 8.71 g --Carbohydrates:176.33 g

56. ONION-MUSHROOM OMELET

Servings: 2   **Cook Time: 10Min**   **Prep Time 15 Min**

INGREDIENTS:
- ✓ 4 eggs, beaten
- ✓ 1 cup mushrooms, sliced
- ✓ 2 tsp olive oil, divided
- ✓ 1 garlic clove, minced
- ✓ Salt and black pepper to taste
- ✓ ¼ cup sliced onions

DIRECTIONS:
- ➢ Warm the olive oil in a frying pan over medium heat
- ➢ Place in garlic, mushrooms, and onions
- ➢ Cook for 6 minutes, stirring often
- ➢ Season with salt and pepper
- ➢ Increase the heat
- ➢ Cook for 3 minutes
- ➢ Remove to a plate. In the same pan
- ➢ Then in the eggs and ensure they are evenly spread
- ➢ Top with the veggies. Slice into wedges and serve.

NUTRITION INFORMATION: Calories 203, Fat 13g, Carbs 7g, Protein 13g

57. SCRAMBLED EGGS WITH VEGETABLES

Servings: 4   **Cook Time: 15 Min**   **Prep Time 15 Min**

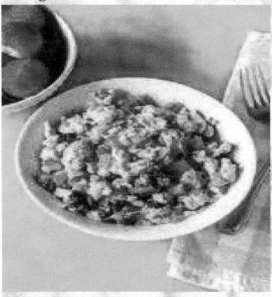

INGREDIENTS:
- ✓ 6 cherry tomatoes, halved
- ✓ 2 tbsp olive oil
- ✓ ½ cup chopped zucchini
- ✓ ½ cup chopped green bell pepper
- ✓ Eggs, beaten 1 shallot, chopped
- ✓ 1 tbsp chopped fresh parsley
- ✓ 1 tbsp chopped fresh basil
- ✓ Salt and black pepper to taste

DIRECTIONS:
- ➢ Warm oil in a pan over medium heat
- ➢ Place in zucchini, salt, black pepper and shallot
- ➢ Cook for 4-5 minutes to sweat the shallot
- ➢ Stir in tomatoes, parsley, and basil
- ➢ Cook for a minute and top with the beaten eggs
- ➢ Lower the heat and cook for 6-7 minutes
- ➢ (Until the eggs are set but not runny)
- ➢ Remove to a platter to serve.

NUTRITION INFORMATION: Calories 205, Fat 15g, Carbs 4g, Protein 12g

58. CITRUS GREEN JUICE

Serving: 1 | **Cook Time: 15 Min** | **Prep Time 5 Min**

INGREDIENTS:
- ½ grapefruit
- ½ lemon
- 3 cups cavolo nero
- 1 cucumber
- ¼ cup fresh parsley leaves
- ¼ pineapple, cut into wedges
- ½ green apple
- 1 tsp grated fresh ginger

DIRECTIONS:
- In a mixer, place the cavolo nero, parsley
- Add cucumber, pineapple, grapefruit, apple, lemon, and ginger
- Pulse until smooth.
- Serve in a tall glass.

NUTRITION INFORMATION: Calories 255, Fat 0.9g, Carbs 60.2g, Protein 9.5g

59. PANCETTA & EGG BENEDICT WITH ARUGULA

Servings: 2 | **Cook Time: 10 Min** | **Prep Time 20 Min**

INGREDIENTS:
- 1 English muffin, toasted and halved
- ¼ cup chopped pancetta
- 2 tsp hollandaise sauce
- 1 cup arugula
- Salt and black pepper to taste
- 2 large eggs

DIRECTIONS:
- Place pancetta in a pan over medium heat
- Cook for 5 minutes until crispy. Remove to a bowl
- In the same pan, crack the eggs and season with salt and pepper
- Cook for 4-5 minutes until the whites are set
- Turn the eggs and cook for an additional minute
- Divide pancetta between muffin halves
- Top each with an egg. Spoon the hollandaise sauce on top
- Sprinkle with arugula to serve

NUTRITION INFORMATION: Calories 173, Fat 7g, Carbs 17g, Protein 11g:

60. LOW CARB SLOPPY JOES

Servings: 4 | **Cook Time: 25 Min** | **Prep Time 5 Min**

INGREDIENTS:
- ½ Tablespoon Cinnamon Chipotle
- Seasoning or ground cinnamon
- Chipotle paste and garlic
- 1 Tablespoon (one Capful)
- Garlic & Spring Onion
- Seasoning or salt, pepper, crushed garlic
- Garlic powder and onion to taste
- 1 Tablespoon yellow mustard
- 1 teaspoon (one packet) powdered stevia
- 2 Tablespoons tomato paste
- 1/2 C diced green bell pepper
- 1 1/2 pounds lean ground beef
- Dash of Desperation
- Salt and Pepper to taste
- 1 Tablespoon of wine vinegar

DIRECTIONS:
- In a frying pan, place the ground beef
- Place it over medium heat on the burner
- When it is frying, split up the larger pieces of beef.
- Cook the meat for about 7 minutes
- Then add the rest of the ingredients (EXCEPT the broth)
- Whisk to mix. Add the water
- Heat up to medium high until combined.
- When the liquid is boiling, reduce the heat to low and let it steam
- (Until the liquid is somewhat reduced)
- Uncovered for around 10-15 minutes.
- Serve warm & have fun!

NUTRITION INFORMATION: 413 kcal--Protein: 46.92 g--Fat: 19.17 g --Carbohydrates:11.08 g

61. BREAKFAST PIZZA WAFFLES

Servings: 2   **Cook Time: 25 Min**   **Prep Time 15 Min**

INGREDIENTS:
- ✓ 4 large Eggs
- ✓ 4 tbsp. Parmesan Cheese
- ✓ 3 tbsp. Almond Flour
- ✓ 1 tbsp. Psyllium Husk Powder
- ✓ 1 tbsp. Bacon Grease(or Butter)
- ✓ 1 tsp. Baking Powder
- ✓ 1 tsp. Italian Seasoning(or spices of choice)
- ✓ Salt and Pepper to Taste
- ✓ 1/2 cup Tomato Sauce
- ✓ 3 oz. Cheddar Cheese
- ✓ 14 slices Pepperoni (optional)

DIRECTIONS:
- ➢ Add all ingredients (except for tomato sauce and cheese) to a container.
- ➢ Use an immersion blender to blend everything.
- ➢ About 30-45 seconds until the mixture thickens.
- ➢ Heat your waffle iron and add half of the mixture to the waffle iron.
- ➢ Let cook until there is little steam coming out of the waffle iron
- ➢ Once done, remove from the iron
- ➢ Repeat with the second half of the mixture
- ➢ Add tomato sauce (1/4 cup per waffle), and cheese (5 oz. per waffle) on the top of each waffle
- ➢ Then, broil for 3-5 minutes in the oven.
- ➢ Optionally add pepperoni to the top of these
- ➢ Once the cheese is melted and starting to crisp on top
- ➢ Remove it from the oven and serve.

NUTRITION INFORMATION: 526 Calories, 45g Fats, 5g Net Carbs, and 29g Protein

62. BREAKFAST BURGER

Servings: 2   **Cook Time: 40 Min**   **Prep Time 20 Min**

INGREDIENTS:
- ✓ 4 oz. Sausage
- ✓ (2 oz. per serving)
- ✓ 2 oz. Pepper Jack Cheese 4 slices Bacon
- ✓ 2 large Eggs
- ✓ 1 tbsp. Butter
- ✓ 1 tbsp. PB Fit Powder Salt and Pepper to Taste

DIRECTIONS:
- ➢ Start by cooking the bacon
- ➢ Lay the strips (however many you want) on a wire rack over a cookie sheet
- ➢ Bake at 400F for 20-25 minutes or until crisp.
- ➢ Mix butter and PB Fit powder in a small container to re-hydrate.
- ➢ Set aside.
- ➢ Form the sausage patties
- ➢ Cook them in a pan over medium-high heat.
- ➢ Flip when the bottom side is browned.
- ➢ Grate the cheese and have it ready.
- ➢ Once the other side of the sausage patty is browned
- ➢ Add cheese and cover with a cloche or lid.
- ➢ Remove sausage patties with melted cheese and set aside
- ➢ Fry an egg over easy in the same pan.
- ➢ Assemble everything: sausage patty, egg, bacon, and rehydrated

NUTRITION INFORMATION: 655 Calories, 56g Fats, 3g Net Carbs, and 30.5g Protein.

63. TEX-MEX SEARED SALMON

Servings: 4 **Cook Time: 15 Min** **Prep Time 5 Min**

INGREDIENTS:

- ✓ 1 Tablespoon (one Capful)
- ✓ Phoenix Sunrise Seasoning or salt, pepper
- ✓ Garlic
- ✓ Cumin
- ✓ Paprika
- ✓ Cayenne, and onion to taste
- ✓ 1 1/2 pounds wild-caught salmon filet (will cook best if you have it at room temp)

DIRECTIONS:

- ➢ Preheat a nonstick pan for 1 min over high heat
- ➢ Swirl seasoning over the salmon during the heating process (NOT on the skin side)
- ➢ Decrease the heat to medium height.
- ➢ Put the fish in the pan and let it cook for about 4-6 minutes depending on the size, seasoned side down
- ➢ When a "crust" has been created from the seasoning and the fish is quickly released from the pan, you will know it's ready to flip.
- ➢ Lower the heat to medium-low
- ➢ Turn the fish down to the side of the skin
- ➢ Cook for about 4-6 more minutes
- ➢ (Less for medium / rare and more for well done)
- ➢ Using a meat thermometer is the safest way to search for crispiness.
- ➢ We cook to 130 degrees
- ➢ Then let it rest for 5 minutes, not overcooked and softly yellow.
- ➢ Withdraw from the flame and serve
- ➢ Fish can slip on to the plate right off the skin

NUTRITION INFORMATION: 244 kcal--Protein: 42.94 g--Fat: 7.91 g Carbohydrates:0.23 g

64. CHILI ZUCCHINI & EGG NESTS

Servings: 4 **Cook Time: 15 Min** **Prep Time 25 Min**

INGREDIENTS:

- ✓ 4 eggs
- ✓ 2 tbsp olive oil
- ✓ 1 lb zucchinis, shredded
- ✓ Salt and black pepper to taste
- ✓ ½ red chili pepper, seeded
- ✓ Minced 2 tbsp parsley, chopped

DIRECTIONS:

- ➢ Preheat the oven to 360 F
- ➢ Combine zucchini, salt, pepper, and *olive oil in a bowl*
- ➢ Form nest shapes with a spoon onto a greased baking sheet
- ➢ Crack an egg into each nest and season with salt, pepper, and chili pepper
- ➢ Bake for 11 minutes
- ➢ Serve topped with parsley.

NUTRITION INFORMATION: Calories 141, Fat 11.6g, Carbs 4.2g, Protein 7g

65. CHARRED SIRLOIN WITH CREAMY HORSERADISH SAUCE

Servings: 4   **Cook Time: 15 Min**   **Prep Time 5 Min**

INGREDIENTS:

- ✓ 1-3 T horseradish (from the jar)
- ✓ 6 Tablespoons low-fat sour cream
- ✓ 1/2 capful
- ✓ (1/2 Tablespoon)
- ✓ Dash of seasoning or salt, pepper, garlic, and onion to taste
- ✓ 1 1/2 pounds sirloin steaks, trimmed & visible fat removed

DIRECTIONS:

- ➤ Preheat the grill to a medium-high temperature.
- ➤ On all sides, season the steak with Splash of Despair Seasoning.
- ➤ Put on the grill and cook on either side for about 5-7 minutes
- ➤ (Based on how thin the steak is and how fried you like your beef)
- ➤ For rare, you'll leave it on less and for medium-well on more.
- ➤ Use a meat thermometer is the perfect way to prepare your steak.
- ➤ When the meat is cooked, mix the sour cream and horseradish to make the sauce
- ➤ To thin the mixture to produce a sauce
- ➤ Add water, one teaspoon at a time. Put aside until done.
- ➤ Let it sit for five min on a cutting board when the meat is done frying, then slice thinly.

NUTRITION INFORMATION: 370 kcal--Protein: 37.03 g--Fat: 22.42 g --Carbohydrates:2.68 g

66. LOW CARB TACO BOWLS

Servings: 4   Cook Time: 20 Min   Prep Time 5 Min

INGREDIENTS:

- ✓ Cauliflower rice
- ✓ 1 large head cauliflower, steamed until soft or frozen ready-to- cook
- ✓ 1 1/2 pounds lean ground beef
- ✓ 2 canned, diced tomatoes (no sugar added, no flavor added)
- ✓ 1-2 capfuls Sunrise or Southwestern Seasoning or low salt taco seasoning

DIRECTIONS:

- ➤ Over medium-high heat, position a large frying pan.
- ➤ In a wide (preferably Nonstick) skillet
- ➤ Add ground beef and sauté for 8- 12 minutes until lightly browned
- ➤ Using a spatula or a cutting implement
- ➤ Cut the bigger bits into smaller parts.
- ➤ Then the tomatoes, then season. Stir to blend.
- ➤ Reduce the heat to low and allow the mixture to simmer
- ➤ (Until the liquid is reduced by 1/2 and pleasant & solid for 5 minutes)
- ➤ Use a food processor or chopping instrument to chop steamed cauliflower into rice-sized bits while cooking
- ➤ Prepare it according to box Directions for using ready-to-cook cauli rice.
- ➤ In a cup, add 1/2 C of cauliflower rice
- ➤ Finish with 1/4 of the meat mixture
- ➤ Top with your favorite condiments and serve sweet.

NUTRITION INFORMATION: 420 kcal-Protein: 46.54 g-Fat: 19.06 g -Carbohydrates:12.24 g

67. TURK ANDSURF BURGERS

Servings: 4 **Prep Time 5 Min**
Cook Time: 20 Min

INGREDIENTS:

- ✓ 1 Tablespoon Skinny Scampi
- ✓ Seasoning or garlic, lemon, parsley, onion, salt, pepper, and celery
- ✓ 8 medium raw shrimp, peeled, deveined, and tails removed (each shrimp should be about 1 oz. each)
- ✓ 1 1/4 pounds (20 oz.) ground turkey

DIRECTIONS:

- ➢ Preheat the 350-degree outdoor bbq.
- ➢ Place the turkey in a large bowl
- ➢ Sprinkle with seasoning and blend well with your hands.
- ➢ Shape the turkey mixture into four different patties.
- ➢ Push two raw shrimps in a heart shape softly into the top of the burger.
- ➢ Place on the grill and cook on both sides for 5-7 minutes until finished
- ➢ (An internal temperature of 165 degrees F is required for Turkey)
- ➢ Remove and enjoy with a fantastic side dish from the barbecue!

NUTRITION INFORMATION: 220 kcal-Protein: 29.54 g-Fat: 11.01 g -Carbohydrates:0.45 g

68. GREEK STUFFED MUSHROOMS WITH FETA

Servings: 4 **Prep Time 10 Min**
Cook Time: 30 Min

INGREDIENTS:

- ✓ Four Portobello mushroom caps (about 4" diameter each) 1/2 C crumbled feta cheese
- ✓ 1/4 teaspoon Dash of Desperation Seasoning (or sea salt and fresh cracked pepper)
- ✓ 1 Tablespoon Mediterranean Seasoning (or basil, oregano, onion, black pepper, rosemary, sage, and parsley)
- ✓ 1 1/2 pounds lean ground beef (or chicken, turkey, or lamb)

DIRECTIONS:

- ➢ In a large dish, combine the meat, seasonings, and feta together
- ➢ Gently blend the mixture with both fingertips
- ➢ Split it into four balls of the same size and leave them in the bowl.
- ➢ In a baking dish, put the mushroom caps (season with a pinch of Desperation's Dash)
- ➢ In a mushroom cap, put a part of the meat mixture
- ➢ Press softly, using your fingertips, so that the mixture fills the cap
- ➢ Repeat the mechanism.
- ➢ Place the baking dish in the oven and cook for 25-30 minutes
- ➢ (Or until the meat's ideal temperature is achieved)
- ➢ Serve warm.

NUTRITION INFORMATION: 411 kcal-Protein: 48.08 g-Fat: 22.54 g -Carbohydrates:0.8 g

69. JALAPENO CHEDDAR WAFFLES

Servings: 2   **Prep Time 10 Min**
Cook Time: 10 Min
INGREDIENTS:

- ✓ 3 OZ. Cream Cheese
- ✓ 3 large Eggs
- ✓ 1 tbsp. Coconut Flour
- ✓ 1 tsp. Psyllium Husk Powder

- ✓ 1 tsp. Baking Powder
- ✓ 1 oz. Cheddar Cheese
- ✓ 1 small Jalapeno
- ✓ Salt and Pepper to Taste

DIRECTIONS:

- ➢ Mix all ingredients except for the cheese and jalapeno using an immersion blender.
- ➢ Once the ingredients are mixed well and smooth, add cheese and jalapeno.

- ➢ Use an immersion blender again to make sure that all of the ingredients are mixed well.
- ➢ Heat your waffle iron, and then pour on the waffle mix. It took about 5-6 minutes in total
- ➢ Top with your favorite toppings, and serve!

NUTRITION INFORMATION: 338 Calories, 28g Fats, 3g Net Carbs, and 16g Protein

70. HAM AND CHEESE STROMBOLI

Servings: 4   **Prep Time 10 Min**
Cook Time: 35 Min

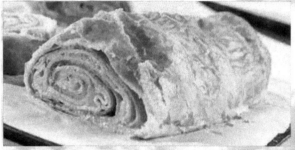

INGREDIENTS:

- ✓ 1 1/4 cups Mozzarella Cheese, shredded
- ✓ 4 tbsp. Almond Flour
- ✓ 3 tbsp. Coconut Flour
- ✓ 1 large Egg
- ✓ 1 tsp. Italian Seasoning
- ✓ 4 oz. Ham
- ✓ 5 oz. Cheddar Cheese
- ✓ Salt and Pepper to Taste

DIRECTIONS:

- ➢ Preheat your oven to 400F and in a microwave or toaster oven, melt your
- ➢ Mozzarella cheese. About 1 minute in the microwave, and 10- second intervals afterward
- ➢ (Or about 10 minutes in an oven), stirring occasionally.
- ➢ Combine almond and coconut flour, as well as your seasonings in a mixing bowl
- ➢ Use salt, pepper, and an Italian blend seasoning.
- ➢ When the mozzarella is melted, place that into your flour mixture and begin working it in.
- ➢ After about a minute, when the cheese has had a chance to cool down
- ➢ Add in your egg and combine everything. It helps to use two utensils here.
- ➢ When everything is combined and you've got a moist dough transfer it to a flat surface with some parchment paper.

- ➢ Lay the second sheet of parchment paper over the dough ball
- ➢ Use a rolling pin or your hand to flatten it out.
- ➢ Use a pizza cutter or knife to cut diagonal lines beginning from the edges of the dough to the center
- ➢ Leave a row of dough untouched about 4 inches wide.
- ➢ Alternate laying ham and cheddar on that uncut stretch of dough.
- ➢ Then lift one section of dough at a time and lay it over the top, covering your filling.
- ➢ Bake it for about 15-20 minutes until you see it has turned a golden brown color.
- ➢ Slice it up and serve!

NUTRITION INFORMATION: 306 Calories, 28g Fats, 7g Net Carbs, and 26g Protein.

71. GRILLED SHRIMP SCAMPI

Servings: 4   **Prep Time 10 Min**
Cook Time: 20 Min
INGREDIENTS:

- ✓ 4 teaspoons Olive Oil
- ✓ 1 3/4 lbs. wild-caught large shrimp, shells removed
- ✓ 1/2 Tablespoons Simply Brilliant Seasoning

DIRECTIONS:

- ➤ In a large pot, add all the ingredients and toss to cover. Let the grill sit until it heats up.
- ➤ Preheat grill to medium-high (about 350 degrees). In a barbecue basket, add the shrimp and put on the barbecue.
- ➤ Cook for 15-20 minutes, tossing it with tongs sometimes
- ➤ When they are dark pink and opaque, you'll know they're thoroughly cooked.
- ➤ Serve chilled or hot.

NUTRITION INFORMATION: 722 kcal-33%-Protein: 29.28 g-Fat: 3.27 g-Carbohydrates: 149.26 g

72. PROTEIN OATCAKES

Serving: 1   **Cook Time: 5 Min**   **Prep Time 10 Min**
INGREDIENTS:

- ✓ 70g oatmeal
- ✓ 15g protein 1 egg white
- ✓ 1/2 cup water
- ✓ 1/2 teaspoon cinnamon
- ✓ 60g curd
- ✓ 1 teaspoon cacao powder
- ✓ 15g sugar

DIRECTIONS

- ➤ Mix the oatmeal, protein, egg white, and water in a bowl.
- ➤ Preheat a saucepan to medium heat.
- ➤ Place the mixture into the saucepan.
- ➤ While waiting, prepare the topping by mixing the curd, cinnamon, and sugar in a second bowl.
- ➤ Remove the oatcake from the saucepan when it becomes golden-brown.
- ➤ Serve on a plate.
- ➤ Add the topping and cocoa powder

NUTRITION INFORMATION: Calories: 440 -Protein: 1.1g -Fiber: 0.8g -Carbohydrates: 6.1g

73. MEDITERRANEAN SALMON

Servings: 4   **Cook Time: 12 Min**   **Prep Time 2 Min**

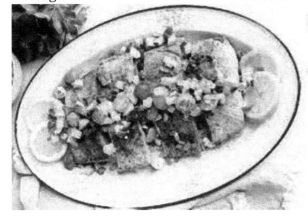

INGREDIENTS:

- ✓ Wild caught salmon - 20 ounces
- ✓ Mediterranean seasoning - 1 tablespoon

DIRECTIONS

- ➤ Grease your pan with nonstick cooking spray and heat over medium-high heat.
- ➤ Meanwhile, season the salmon.
- ➤ With the seasoned side down, place the salmon in the pan and allow it to sear for about 2 minutes.
- ➤ Flip and lower the heat to medium.
- ➤ Cover the pan and cook for extra 6 minutes, or until the salmon is well cooked.
- ➤ Then serve.

NUTRITION INFORMATION: 188 -Fats: 8.8g -Carbs: 0g -Fiber: 0g -Sugar: 0g -Protein: 27.5g

74. CITRUS FLOUNDER

Servings: 4   **Cook Time: 10 Min**   **Prep Time 5 Min**

INGREDIENTS:

- ✓ 1 3/4 pounds lounder filets -
- ✓ 4 teaspoons Lemon oil (Olive oil and lemon zest)

- ✓ 1-2 tablespoons Citrus dill seasoning (or use any other seasoning you like)

DIRECTIONS

- ➤ Heat the oil over medium-high heat with a nonstick pan
- ➤ Add the fish fillets and sprinkle over with the seasoning

- ➤ Cook each side of the fillets for about 2 minutes, or until it becomes opaque and flaky.
- ➤ Serve.

NUTRITION INFORMATION: Calories:189 -Fats: 6.5g -Carbs: 0g -Fiber: 0g- Sugar: 0g - Protein: 30.7g

75. LEMON RADISHES

Servings: 4   **Cook Time: 30 Min**   **Prep Time 5 Min**

INGREDIENTS:

- ✓ Red radish halves - 4 cup
- ✓ 2 teaspoons of olive oil

- ✓ Citrus dill seasoning - 1/2 tablespoon
- ✓ Freshly squeezed lemon - 1/2 tablespoon

DIRECTIONS

- ➤ Preheat your oven to 350.
- ➤ Trim the radish and cut into half and equal sizes.
- ➤ Add and toss all ingredients in a bowl until well combined.

- ➤ Place the mixture in oven-safe dish and cook/roast for 30 minutes
- ➤ Then serve

NUTRITION INFORMATION: Calories: 39 Fats: 2.4g Carbs: 3.9g Fiber: 1.9g Sugar: 2.2g Protein: 0.8g

76. MAHI MAHI BASIL BUTTER

Servings: 4   **Cook Time: 15Min**   **Prep Time 5 Min**

INGREDIENTS:

- ✓ Butter - 4 tablespoons
- ✓ Garlic and spring onion seasoning (or use parsley, chopped garlic, and chives) - 1 tablespoon
- ✓ Fresh basil leaves (chopped) - 2 tablespoons
- ✓ Fresh lemon juice - 1 tablespoon

- ✓ Fresh mahi mahi filets (wild caught, or you can use flaky white fish, thinly sliced chicken, or shrimp) - 2 pounds
- ✓ Seasoning (or use salt, garlic, and pepper)

DIRECTIONS

- ➤ With your sauce pot, melt the butter over low heat.
- ➤ Add the garlic seasoning, lemon, and basil.
- ➤ Stir mixture to combine well and set it aside
- ➤ Keep the mixture warm.
- ➤ Grease your pan with nonstick cooking spray and heat it up over medium high heat.
- ➤ Sprinkle over with the seasoning.

- ➤ Once the pan is heated up
- ➤ Add the fish and cook each side for about 3 minutes
- ➤ (Or until the fish is fully cooked)
- ➤ Remove from the pan and drizzle over with the melted butter.
- ➤ Then serve.

NUTRITION INFORMATION: Calories:269 -Fats: 12.9g -Carbs: 0.1g -Fiber: 0g -Sugar: 0.1g -Protein: 36.3g

77. FISH TACOS

Servings: 4   **Cook Time: 15Min**   **Prep Time 15 Min**

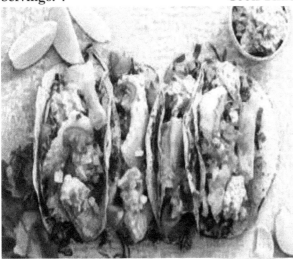

INGREDIENTS:
- ✓ Cod (or haddock, wild caught) - 1 3/4 lbs.
- ✓ Taco seasoning (low sodium) - 1 tablespoon
- ✓ Roasted garlic oil (Olive oil and fresh garlic) - 4 teaspoons
- ✓ Preferred taco condiment

DIRECTIONS
- ➢ Pat dry the fish and cut it into 1-inch chunks.
- ➢ Sprinkle over with the seasoning and gently
- ➢ Toss thoroughly to coat completely.
- ➢ Add the oil over a nonstick pan and heat over medium-high heat.
- ➢ Add the fish and cook for additional 12 minutes
- ➢ (Or until the fish breaks apart into flakes and turns opaque)
- ➢ Then serve with the condiments.

NUTRITION INFORMATION: 151 -Fats: 1.3g -Carbs: 0.2g -Fiber: 0.1g -Sugar: 0g -Protein: 32.5g

78. GARLIC SEASONED ZOODLES

Servings: 4   **Cook Time: 5Min**   **Prep Time 5 Min**

INGREDIENTS:
- ✓ Roasted garlic oil (or any other oil you like) - 1tablespoon
- ✓ Zucchini noodles - 6 cups
- ✓ Garlic and spring onion seasoning
- ✓ (Or use a mixture of fresh chopped garlic, pepper, and salt) - 1/2 tablespoon
- ✓ Pinch of salt and pepper

DIRECTIONS:
- ➢ With your pan, heat the oil over medium-high heat.
- ➢ Add the noodles and sprinkle over with the seasoning.
- ➢ Cook for about 3 minutes. Toss occasionally.
- ➢ Season with a pinch of pepper and salt.
- ➢ Serve.

NUTRITION INFORMATION: Calories:57 -Fats: 3.7g -Carbs: 5.7g -Fiber: 1.9g -Sugar: 2.9g -Protein: 2.1g

79. CAULIFLOWER SCALLOPS

Servings: 4   **Cook Time: 25Min**   **Prep Time 5 Min**

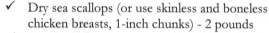

INGREDIENTS:

- ✓ Dry sea scallops (or use skinless and boneless chicken breasts, 1-inch chunks) - 2 pounds
- ✓ Seasoning (or use salt & pepper) - 1 teaspoon
- ✓ 4 teaspoon Olive Oil
- ✓ Diced tomatoes (no added sugar) - 3 cup
- ✓ Cajun seasoning (or use any blackening seasoning) 2 teaspoons
- ✓ Fresh lime juice - 2 tablespoon
- ✓ Cooked cauliflower rice - 3 cup
- ✓ To garnish, use sliced scallion greens and fresh cilantro

DIRECTIONS:

- ➢ Pat dry the scallops with paper towel
- ➢ Season with pepper and salt.
- ➢ Add the oil to a pan and heat over medium-high heat.
- ➢ Add the scallops to the pan and cook on each side for about 2 minutes, or until they turn brown.
- ➢ For chicken, cook for 7 minutes, or until it turns brown.
- ➢ Remove the scallops and set them aside.

- ➢ Add the seasonings and tomatoes to the pan.
- ➢ Bring mixture to a boil and scrape all the brown bits from the bottom of the pan.
- ➢ Once it starts to boil, lower heat to medium and simmer for about 10 minutes.
- ➢ Return the scallops to the pan
- ➢ Cook for extra 5 minutes, or until it is fully cooked
- ➢ For chicken, allow it to cook for about 15 minutes.
- ➢ Serve.

NUTRITION INFORMATION: Calories: 258 -Fats: 6.4g -Carbs: 13.9g -Fiber: 3.5g-Sugar: 5.4g -Protein: 36g

80. GRILLED MEDITERRANEAN LAMB BURGERS

Servings: 4   **Cook Time: 15Min**   **Prep Time 5 Min**

INGREDIENTS:

- ✓ Ground lamb (you can use other ground meat) - 1 1/4 lbs.
- ✓ Mediterranean seasoning (or use a mixture of basil, oregano, marjoram, onion, garlic, and parsley) - 1 tablespoon

- ✓ Seasoning (or use a mixture of onion, garlic, salt, & pepper) - 1/2 tsp.

DIRECTIONS:

- ➢ Preheat your grill to medium-high heat.
- ➢ Mix all the ingredients in a bowl.
- ➢ Equally divide the mixture into 4 portions.
- ➢ Press the portions into 1/3-inch thick patties.

- ➢ Place the patties on the grill and cook each side for about 5 minutes.
- ➢ Remove from heat and serve.

NUTRITION INFORMATION: Calories: 313 -Fats: 21.7g -Carbs: 0g -Fiber: 0g -Sugar: 0g -Protein: 27.4g

81. MINI PANCAKE DONUTS

Servings: 8   **Cook Time: 25 Min**   **Prep Time 5 Min**

INGREDIENTS:
- ✓ 3 OZ. Cream Cheese 3 large Eggs
- ✓ 4 tbsp. Almond Flour
- ✓ 1 tbsp. Coconut Flour
- ✓ 1 tsp. Baking Powder
- ✓ 1 tsp. Vanilla Extract
- ✓ 4 tbsp. Erythritol
- ✓ 10 drops Liquid Stevia

DIRECTIONS:
- ➢ Stick all of the ingredients inside of a container and mix them using an immersion blender.
- ➢ Make sure that you continue to mix everything for about 45-60 seconds
- ➢ (Ensuring a smooth batter that's slightly thickened)
- ➢ Heat donut maker and spray with coconut oil to ensure non-stick properties
- ➢ Pour batter into each well of the donut maker, filling about 90% of the way.
- ➢ Let cook for 3 minutes on one side
- ➢ Then flip and cook for an additional 2 minutes
- ➢ This is more time than my donut maker tells me to cook them
- ➢ Remove donuts from the donut maker and set them aside to cool
- ➢ Repeat the process with the rest of the batter.
- ➢ This makes a total of 22 Mini Pancake Donuts.

NUTRITION INFORMATION: 32 Calories, 7g Fats, 0.4g Net Carbs, and 4g Protein.

82. WHITE PIZZA WITH BROCCOLI CRUST

Servings: 2   **Cook Time: 35 Min**   **Prep Time 10 Min**

INGREDIENTS:
- ✓ 2 1/2 cups broccoli (riced)
- ✓ 1 egg
- ✓ 1/3 cup + ¾ cup shredded mozzarella cheese (low-fat)
- ✓ 1/4 cup grated Parmesan cheese
- ✓ 1/2 tsp. Italian seasoning
- ✓ 1/2 cup ricotta cheese (part-skim)
- ✓ 1/4 tsp. red pepper flakes
- ✓ 1 garlic clove (minced)
- ✓ 1/2 cup broccoli florets (chopped)

DIRECTIONS:
- ➢ Preheat oven to 400°F.
- ➢ Cook broccoli in a microwave-safe tray and then cover it (about 3 minutes).
- ➢ Once cooled, transfer "rice" to a cheesecloth or clean, thin dishtowel, and squeeze out as much liquid as possible.
- ➢ Take a bowl and mix in broccoli, egg, one-third cup Mozzarella cheese, Parmesan cheese, and Italian seasoning, and combine well.
- ➢ Form mixture into a square pizza (1/3 inch thick) onto a baking sheet. Bake until edges are brown (15-20 minutes).
- ➢ Meanwhile, take a bowl and combine ricotta, red pepper flakes, and garlic
- ➢ Then spread this ricotta mixture onto broccoli crust
- ➢ Sprinkle with the remaining mozzarella, and top with broccoli. Bake for an additional until cheese is melted (about 5- 10 minutes)

NUTRITION INFORMATION: 279 kcal-protein:23.85 g-Fat: 16.72 g-Carbohydrates: 9.51 g

83. VEGETABLE EGG BAKE

Servings: 4   **Cook Time: 30 Min**   **Prep Time 10 Min**

INGREDIENTS:

- ✓ ½ cup whole milk 8 eggs
- ✓ 1 cup spinach, chopped
- ✓ 4 oz canned artichokes, chopped
- ✓ 1 garlic clove, minced
- ✓ ½ cup Parmesan cheese, crumbled
- ✓ 1 tsp oregano, dried
- ✓ 1 tsp Jalapeño pepper, minced
- ✓ Salt to taste 2 tsp olive oil

DIRECTIONS:

- ➢ Preheat oven to 360 F
- ➢ Warm the olive oil in a skillet over medium heat
- ➢ Then sauté garlic and spinach for 3 minutes
- ➢ Beat the eggs in a bowl.
- ➢ Stir in artichokes, milk, Parmesan cheese, oregano, jalapeño pepper, and salt
- ➢ Add in spinach mixture and toss to combine
- ➢ Transfer to a greased baking dish and bake for 20 minutes
- ➢ (Until golden and bubbling)
- ➢ Slice into wedges and serve.

NUTRITION INFORMATION: Calories 190, Fat 14g, Carbs 5g, Protein 10g

84. CREAMY MASHED CAULIFLOWER AND GRAVY

Servings: 4   **Cook Time: 20 Min**   **Prep Time 10 Min**

INGREDIENTS:

- ✓ 4 cups cauliflower florets
- ✓ 1/4 cup cream cheese (low-fat, softened)
- ✓ 1 tbsp. butter (unsalted, melted)
- ✓ 1 clove garlic
- ✓ 1 tbsp. rosemary
- ✓ 1/4 tsp. salt
- ✓ 1/4 tsp. black pepper
- ✓ 3 tbsp. gravy mix or mushroom gravy mix
- ✓ ¾ cup cold water

DIRECTIONS:

- ➢ Put water in a pot and let it boil
- ➢ Then, boil cauliflower, until easily pierced with a fork (about 10 minutes)
- ➢ Drain and let it cool slightly.
- ➢ Add the cauliflower and the remaining ingredients into a blender and mix until smooth.
- ➢ Prepare gravy according to package directions

NUTRITION INFORMATION: 90 kcal-Protein: 3.75 g-Fat: 5.76 g -Carbohydrates: 7.51 g

85. AWESOME TUNA SALAD

Servings: 2   **Cook Time: 20 Min**   **Prep Time 10 Min**

INGREDIENTS:

- ✓ ½ iceberg lettuce, torn
- ✓ ¼ endive, chopped
- ✓ 1 tomato, cut into wedges
- ✓ 2 tbsp olive oil
- ✓ 5 oz canned tuna in water, flaked
- ✓ 4 black olives, pitted and sliced
- ✓ 1 tbsp lemon juice
- ✓ Salt and black pepper to taste

DIRECTIONS:

- ➢ In a salad bowl, mix olive oil, lemon juice, salt, and pepper
- ➢ Add in lettuce, endive, and tuna and toss to coat
- ➢ Top with black olives and tomato wedges
- ➢ Serve.

NUTRITION INFORMATION: Calories 260, Fat 18g, Carbs 3g, Protein 11g

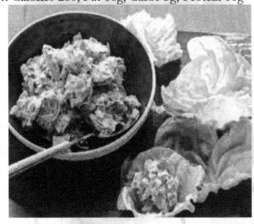

86. ROASTED VEGGIE WITH PEANUT SAUCE

Servings: 4   **Cook Time: 30 Min**   **Prep Time 10 Min**

INGREDIENTS:
- ✓ 1 1/2 cups cauliflower florets
- ✓ 1 1/2 cups broccoli florets
- ✓ 1 1/2 cups red cabbage (cut into bite-sized pieces)
- ✓ 1 bell pepper (remove seeds and membranes, chopped)
- ✓ 1/4 tsp. salt and black pepper (each)
- ✓ 3 1/2 lbs. firm tofu (sliced 1/4 - 1/2 inch blocks)
- ✓ 2 tbsp. peanut butter (powdered)
- ✓ 3 tbsp. water
- ✓ 1/2 tbsp. sambal

DIRECTIONS:
- ➤ Preheat oven to 400°F.
- ➤ Spread all of the vegetables evenly on a lightly greased baking sheet
- ➤ Season with salt and black pepper.
- ➤ Roast veggies until caramelized yet tender
- ➤ Take a pan and sear tofu in a single layer in batches
- ➤ (Until both sides are golden brown)
- ➤ To make a peanut sauce, take a bowl
- ➤ Whisk together the powdered peanut butter, water, and sambal
- ➤ To serve, place tofu in a bowl, top with roasted veggies, and drizzle with peanut sauce

NUTRITION INFORMATION: 623 kcal-Protein: 64.98 g-Fat: 36.3 g -Carbohydrates: 24.08 g

87. SHRIMP & AVOCADO SALAD

Servings: 4   **Cook Time: 15 Min**   **Prep Time 10 Min**

INGREDIENTS:
- ✓ 2 tbsp olive oil
- ✓ 1 tbsp lemon juice
- ✓ 1 yellow bell pepper, sliced
- ✓ 1 Romano lettuce, torn
- ✓ 1 avocado, chopped Salt to taste
- ✓ 1 lb shrimp, peeled and deveined
- ✓ 1 cups cherry tomatoes, halved

DIRECTIONS:
- ➤ Preheat grill pan over high heat
- ➤ Drizzle the shrimp with some olive oil and arrange them on the preheated grill pan
- ➤ Sear for 5 minutes on both sides until pink and cooked through
- ➤ Let cool completely
- ➤ In a serving plate, arrange the lettuce
- ➤ Top with bell pepper, shrimp, avocado, and cherry tomatoes
- ➤ In a bowl, add the lemon juice, salt, and olive oil
- ➤ Whisk to combine
- ➤ Drizzle the dressing over the salad and serve immediately

NUTRITION INFORMATION: Calories 380, Fat 24g, Carbs 23g, Protein 25g

88. CHEESY BROCCOLI BITES

Servings: 4   **Cook Time: 45 Min**   **Prep Time 10 Min**

INGREDIENTS:
- ➤ 6 cups frozen broccoli (steamed-in-bag)
- ➤ 1/4 cup thinly sliced scallions
- ➤ 4 large eggs
- ➤ 2 cups cottage cheese (1%)
- ➤ 1 1/4 cup shredded mozzarella cheese (low-fat)
- ➤ 1/4 cup parmesan cheese
- ➤ 2 tsp. olive oil
- ➤ 1 tsp. garlic powder
- ➤ 1/4 tsp. salt Cooking spray

DIRECTIONS:
- ➤ Preheat oven to 375°F.
- ➤ Cook broccoli according to package directions.
- ➤ Once cooked, add broccoli to the food processor and blend until finely chopped
- ➤ Then, add scallions, eggs, cottage cheese, mozzarella, parmesan, olive oil, garlic
- ➤ Salt to broccoli, and blend until well combined.
- ➤ Scoop mixture into 20 to 24 slots of two lightly greased muffin tins
- ➤ Bake until the filling is set and golden brown (about 25-30 minutes).

NUTRITION INFORMATION: 317 kcal-Protein: 34.05 g-Fat: 13.7 g -Carbohydrates: 18.01 g

89. ONE-PAN EGGPLANT QUINOA

Servings: 4   **Cook Time: 25 Min**   **Prep Time 10 Min**

INGREDIENTS:

- ✓ 2 tbsp olive oil
- ✓ 1 shallot, chopped
- ✓ 2 garlic cloves, minced
- ✓ 1 tomato, chopped
- ✓ 1 cup quinoa
- ✓ 1 eggplant, cubed

- ✓ 2 tbsp basil, chopped
- ✓ ¼ cup green olives, pitted and chopped
- ✓ ½ cup feta cheese, crumbled
- ✓ 1 cup canned garbanzo beans, drained and rinsed
- ✓ Salt and black pepper to taste

DIRECTIONS:

- ➤ Warm the olive oil in a skillet over medium heat
- ➤ Sauté garlic, shallot, and eggplant for 4-5 minutes until tender
- ➤ Pour in quinoa and 2 cups of water

- ➤ Season with salt and pepper and bring to a boil
- ➤ Reduce the heat to low and cook for 15 minutes
- ➤ Stir in olives, feta cheese, and garbanzo beans
- ➤ Serve topped with basil.

NUTRITION INFORMATION: Calories 320, Fat 12g, Carbs 45g, Protein 12g

90. CAULIFLOWER LATKES

Servings: 2   **Cook Time: 30 Min**   **Prep Time 10 Min**

INGREDIENTS:

- ✓ 2 packets rosemary crackers (ground to a flour-like consistency)
- ✓ 2 1/2 cups cauliflower (riced)
- ✓ 1 egg
- ✓ 1/4 cup onion (diced)
- ✓ 1/4 tsp. salt
- ✓ 1/4 tsp. black pepper
- ✓ Cooking spray
- ✓ 1/2 cup green onion (sliced)
- ✓ 1 cup Greek yogurt (low-fat)

DIRECTIONS:

- ➤ Take a bowl and combine the first six ingredients.
- ➤ Heat a lightly greased pan over medium heat
- ➤ Take one-third of the cauliflower mixture and divided it into two mounds on the pan
- ➤ Flatten each mound into a circular patty (about 1/4 inch thick)

- ➤ Cook them they get a golden brown color (about 3-5 minutes per side)
- ➤ Repeat with the remaining mixture.
- ➤ Garnish with green onions and serve with Greek yogurt.

NUTRITION INFORMATION: 73 kcal-Protein: 4.95 g-Fat: 3.54 g -Carbohydrates: 6.5 g

91. ARUGULA & GORGONZOLA SALAD

Servings: 4   **Cook Time: 10 Min**   **Prep Time 10 Min**

INGREDIENTS:

- ✓ 3 tbsp olive oil
- ✓ 1 cucumber, cubed
- ✓ 15 oz canned garbanzo beans, drained
- ✓ 3 oz black olives, pitted and sliced
- ✓ 1 Roma tomato, slivered
- ✓ ¼ cup red onion, chopped
- ✓ 5 cups arugula Salt to taste
- ✓ ½ cup Gorgonzola cheese, crumbled
- ✓ 1 tbsp lemon juice
- ✓ 2 tbsp parsley, chopped

DIRECTIONS:

- ➢ Place the arugula in a salad bowl
- ➢ Add in garbanzo beans, cucumber, olives, tomato, and onion and mix to combine
- ➢ In another small bowl, whisk the lemon juice, olive oil, and salt
- ➢ Drizzle the dressing over the salad
- ➢ Sprinkle with gorgonzola cheese to serve.

NUTRITION INFORMATION: Calories 280, Fat 17g, Carbs 25g, Protein 10g

92. GREEK-STYLE PASTA SALAD

Servings: 4   **Cook Time: 15 Min**   **Prep Time 10 Min**

INGREDIENTS:

- ✓ 2 tbsp olive oil
- ✓ 16 oz fusilli pasta
- ✓ 1 yellow bell pepper, cubed
- ✓ 1 green bell pepper, cubed
- ✓ Salt and black pepper to taste
- ✓ 3 tomatoes, cubed 1 red onion, sliced
- ✓ 2 cups feta cheese, crumbled
- ✓ ¼ cup lemon juice
- ✓ 1 tbsp lemon zest, grated
- ✓ 1 cucumber, cubed
- ✓ 1 cup Kalamata olives, pitted and sliced

DIRECTIONS:

- ➢ Cook the fusilli pasta in boiling salted water until "al dente", 8-10 minutes
- ➢ Drain and set asite to cool
- ➢ In a bowl, whisk together olive oil, lemon zst, lemon juice, and salt.
- ➢ Add in bell peppers, tomatoes, onion, feta cheese
- ➢ Then cucumber, olives, and pasta and toss to combine
- ➢ Serve immediately.

NUTRITION INFORMATION: Calories 420, Fat 18g, Carbs 50g, Protein 15g

93. ORANGE RICOTTA PANCAKES

Serving: 1   **Cook Time: 5 Min**   **Prep Time 10 Min**

INGREDIENTS:

- ¾ cup all-purpose flour
- 1/2 tablespoon baking powder
- 2 teaspoons sugar
- 1/2 teaspoon salt
- 3 separated eggs
- 1 cup fresh ricotta
- ¾ cup whole milk
- 1/2 teaspoon pure vanilla extract
- 1 large ripe orange

DIRECTIONS:

- Mix the flour, baking powder, sugar in a large bowl.
- Add a pinch of salt.
- In a separate bowl, whisk egg yolk, ricotta, milk, orange zest, and orange juice.
- Add some vanilla extract for additional flavor.
- Followed by the dry ingredients to the ricotta mixture and mix adequately.
- Stir the egg white in a different bowl, and then gently fold it in the ricotta mixture.

- Preheat saucepan to medium heat and brush with some butter until evenly spread.
- Use a measuring cup to drop the batter onto the saucepan, ensure the pan is not crowded.
- Allow cooking for 2 minutes.
- Flip the food when you notice the edges begin to set, and bubbles form in the center. Cook the meat for another 1 to 2 minutes, serve

NUTRITION INFORMATION: Calories 160 -Fat: 10g -Carbohydrate: 28g -Protein: 6g

94. CHEESY THYME WAFFLES

Servings: 2   **Cook Time: 10 Min**   **Prep Time 15 Min**

INGREDIENTS:

- ½ cup mozzarella cheese, finely shredded
- ¼ cup Parmesan cheese ¼ large head cauliflower
- ½ cup collard greens
- 1 large egg
- 1 stalk green onion
- ½ tablespoon olive oil
- ½ teaspoon garlic powder
- ¼ teaspoon salt
- ½ tablespoon sesame seed
- 1 teaspoon fresh thyme, chopped
- ¼ teaspoon ground black pepper

DIRECTIONS:

- Put cauliflower, collard greens
- Spring onion and thyme in a food processor and pulse until smooth
- Dish out the mixture in a bowl and stir in rest of the ingredients

- Heat a waffle iron and transfer the mixture evenly over the griddle
- Cook until a waffle is formed and dish out in a serving platter

NUTRITION INFORMATION: Calories: 144 Carbs: 8.5g Fats: 9.4g Proteins: 9.3g Sodium: 435mg Sugar: 3g

95. CHICKPEA AND ZUCCHINI SALAD

Servings: 3   **Cook Time: 0 Min**   **Prep Time 10 Min**

INGREDIENTS:
- ✓ ¼ cup balsamic vinegar
- ✓ 1/3 cup chopped basil leaves
- ✓ 1 tablespoon of capers, drained and chopped
- ✓ ½ cup crumbled feta cheese
- ✓ 1 can chickpeas, drained
- ✓ 1 garlic clove, chopped
- ✓ ½ cup Kalamata olives, chopped
- ✓ 1/3 cup of olive oil
- ✓ ½ cup sweet onion, chopped
- ✓ ½ tsp oregano
- ✓ 1 pinch of red pepper flakes, crushed
- ✓ ¾ cup red bell pepper, chopped
- ✓ 1 tablespoon chopped rosemary
- ✓ 2 cups of zucchini, diced
- ✓ Salt and pepper, to taste

DIRECTIONS:
- ➢ Combine the vegetables in a bowl and cover well.
- ➢ Serve at room temperature
- ➢ But for best results, refrigerate the bowl for a few hours before serving, to allow the flavors to blend.

NUTRITION INFORMATION: Calories:258 Fat:12g Carbohydrates:19g Protein:5.6g Sodium:686mg

96. PROVENCAL ARTICHOKE SALAD

Servings: 3   **Cook Time: 5 Min**   **Prep Time 15 Min**

INGREDIENTS:
- ✓ 9 oz artichoke hearts
- ✓ 1 teaspoon of chopped basil
- ✓ 2 garlic cloves, chopped 1 lemon zest
- ✓ 1 tablespoon olives, chopped
- ✓ 1 tablespoon of olive oil
- ✓ ½ chopped onion
- ✓ 1 pinch, ½ teaspoon of salt
- ✓ 2 tomatoes, chopped
- ✓ 3 tablespoons of water
- ✓ ½ glass of white wine
- ✓ Salt and pepper, to taste

DIRECTIONS:
- ➢ Heat the oil in a skillet. Sauté the onion and garlic
- ➢ Cook until the onions are translucent and season with a pinch of salt
- ➢ Pour in the white wine and simmer until the wine is reduced by half.
- ➢ Add the chopped tomatoes, artichoke hearts and water
- ➢ Simmer then add the lemon zest and about ½ teaspoon of salt.
- ➢ Cover and cook for about 6 minutes.
- ➢ Add the olives and basil. Season well and enjoy!

NUTRITION INFORMATION: Calories:147 Fat:13g Carbohydrates:18g Protein:4g Sodium:689mg

97. BULGARIAN SALAD

Servings: 2 **Cook Time: 20Min** **Prep Time 10 Min**

INGREDIENTS:
- ✓ 2 cups of bulgur
- ✓ 1 tablespoon of butter
- ✓ 1 cucumber, cut into pieces
- ✓ ¼ cup dill
- ✓ ¼ cup black olives, cut in half
- ✓ 1 tablespoon
- ✓ 2 teaspoons of olive oil
- ✓ 4 cups of water
- ✓ 2 teaspoons of red wine vinegar salt, to taste

DIRECTIONS:
- ➤ In a saucepan, toast the bulgur on a mixture of butter and olive oil
- ➤ Leave to cook until the bulgur is golden brown and begins to crack.
- ➤ Add water and season with salt
- ➤ Wrap everything and simmer for about 20 minutes or until the bulgur is tender.
- ➤ In a bowl, mix the cucumber pieces with the olive oil, dill, red wine vinegar and black olives
- ➤ Mix everything well.
- ➤ It combines cucumber and bulgur.

NUTRITION INFORMATION: Calories:386 Fat:14g Carbohydrates:55g Protein:9g Sodium:545mg

98. FALAFEL SALAD BOWL

Servings: 2 **Cook Time: 5 Min** **Prep Time 15 Min**

INGREDIENTS:
- ✓ 1 tablespoon of chili garlic sauce
- ✓ 1 tablespoon of garlic and dill sauce
- ✓ 1 pack of vegetarian falafels
- ✓ 1 box of humus
- ✓ 2 tablespoons of lemon juice
- ✓ 1 tablespoon of pitted kalamata olives
- ✓ 1 tablespoon of extra virgin olive oil
- ✓ ¼ cup onion, diced
- ✓ 2 cups of chopped parsley
- ✓ 2 cups of crisp pita
- ✓ 1 pinch of salt
- ✓ 1 tablespoon of tahini sauce
- ✓ ½ cup diced tomato

DIRECTIONS:
- ➤ Cook the prepared falafels. Put it aside.
- ➤ Prepare the salad. Mix the parsley, onion, tomato, lemon juice, olive oil and salt
- ➤ Throw it all out and put everything aside.
- ➤ Transfer everything to the serving bowls.
- ➤ Add the parsley and cover with humus and falafel.
- ➤ Sprinkle bowl with tahini sauce, chili garlic sauce and dill sauce.
- ➤ Upon serving, add the lemon juice and mix the salad well
- ➤ Serve with pita bread on the side.

NUTRITION INFORMATION: Calories:561 Fat:11g Carbohydrates:60.1g Protein:18.5g Sodium:944mg

99. EASY GREEK SALAD

Servings: 2   **Cook Time: 0 Min**   **Prep Time 15 Min**

INGREDIENTS:
- ✓ 4 oz Greek feta cheese, cubed
- ✓ 5 cucumbers, cut lengthwise
- ✓ 1 teaspoon of honey
- ✓ 1 lemon, chewed and grated
- ✓ 1 cup kalamata olives, pitted and halved
- ✓ ¼ cup extra virgin olive oil
- ✓ 1 onion, sliced
- ✓ 1 teaspoon of oregano
- ✓ 1 pinch of fresh oregano (for garnish)
- ✓ 12 tomatoes, quartered
- ✓ ¼ cup red wine vinegar salt and pepper, to taste

DIRECTIONS:
- ➢ In a bowl, soak the onions in salted water for 15 minutes.
- ➢ In a large bowl, combine the honey, lemon juice, lemon peel, oregano, salt and pepper.
- ➢ Mix everything.
- ➢ Gradually add the olive oil, beating as you do, until the oil emulsifies
- ➢ Add the olives and tomatoes. Put it right. Add the cucumbers
- ➢ Drain the onions soaked in salted water and add them to the salad mixture
- ➢ Top the salad with fresh oregano and feta
- ➢ Dash with olive oil and season with pepper, to taste.

NUTRITION INFORMATION: Calories:292 Fat:17g Carbohydrates:12g Protein:6g Sodium:743mg

100.   ARUGULA SALAD WITH FIGS AND WALNUTS

Servings: 2   **Cook Time: 10 Min**   **Prep Time 15 Min**

INGREDIENTS:
- ✓ 5 oz arugula
- ✓ 1 carrot, scraped
- ✓ 1/8 teaspoon of cayenne pepper
- ✓ 3 oz of goat cheese, crumbled
- ✓ 1 can salt-free chickpeas, drained
- ✓ ½ cup dried figs, cut into wedges
- ✓ 1 teaspoon of honey
- ✓ 3 tablespoons of olive oil
- ✓ 2 teaspoons of balsamic vinegar
- ✓ ½ walnuts cut in half salt, to taste

DIRECTIONS:
- ➢ Preheat the oven to 175 degrees
- ➢ In a baking dish, combine the nuts, 1 tablespoon of olive oil
- ➢ Add cayenne pepper and 1/8 teaspoon of salt
- ➢ Transfer the baking sheet in the oven and bake it until the nuts are golden
- ➢ Set it aside when you are done.
- ➢ In a bowl, incorporate the honey, balsamic vinegar, 2 tablespoons of oil and ¾ teaspoon of salt.
- ➢ In a large bowl, combine the arugula, carrot and figs
- ➢ Then nuts and goat cheese and drizzle with balsamic honey vinaigrette
- ➢ Make sure you cover everything

NUTRITION INFORMATION: Calories:403 Fat:9g Carbohydrates:35g Protein:13g Sodium:844mg

101. MEDITERRANEAN BURRITO

Servings: 3   **Cook Time: 0 Min**   **Prep Time 10 Min**

INGREDIENTS:

- ✓ 1 wheat tortillas
- ✓ 2 oz. red kidney beans, canned, drained
- ✓ 2 tablespoons hummus
- ✓ 2 teaspoons tahini sauce 1 cucumber
- ✓ 2 lettuce leaves
- ✓ 1 tablespoon lime juice
- ✓ 1 teaspoon olive oil
- ✓ 1/2 teaspoon dried oregano

DIRECTIONS:

- ➢ Mash the red kidney beans until you get a puree.
- ➢ Then spread the wheat tortillas with beans mash from one side.
- ➢ Add hummus and tahini sauce.
- ➢ Cut the cucumber into the wedges and place them over tahini sauce.
- ➢ Then add lettuce leaves.
- ➢ Make the dressing: mix up together olive oil, dried oregano, and lime juice.
- ➢ Drizzle the lettuce leaves with the dressing
- ➢ Wrap the wheat tortillas in the shape of burritos.

NUTRITION INFORMATION: Calories: 288 Fat: 10.2 Fiber: 14.6 Carbs: 38.2 Protein: 12.5

102. SWEET POTATO BACON MASH

Servings: 4   **Cook Time: 20 Min**   **Prep Time 10 Min**

INGREDIENTS:

- ✓ 3 sweet potatoes, peeled
- ✓ 4 oz. bacon, chopped
- ✓ 1 cup chicken stock
- ✓ 1 tablespoon butter
- ✓ 1 teaspoon salt
- ✓ 2 oz. Parmesan, grated

DIRECTIONS:

- ➢ Dice sweet potato and put it in the pan.
- ➢ Add chicken stock and close the lid.
- ➢ Boil the vegetables for until they are soft.
- ➢ After this, drain the chicken stock.
- ➢ Mash the sweet potato with the help of the potato masher
- ➢ Than add grated cheese and butter.
- ➢ Mix up together salt and chopped bacon
- ➢ Fry the mixture until it is crunchy (10-15 minutes).
- ➢ Add cooked bacon in the mashed sweet potato
- ➢ Mix up with the help of the spoon.
- ➢ It is recommended to serve the meal warm or hot.

NUTRITION INFORMATION: Calories: 304 Fat: 18.1 Fiber: 2.9 Carbs: 18.8 Protein: 17

103. PROSCIUTTO WRAPPED MOZZARELLA BALLS

Servings: 4   **Cook Time: 10 Min**   **Prep Time 10 Min**

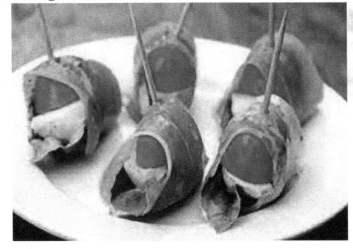

INGREDIENTS:

- ✓ 8 Mozzarella balls, cherry size
- ✓ 4 oz. bacon, sliced
- ✓ 1/4 teaspoon ground black pepper
- ✓ ¾ teaspoon dried rosemary
- ✓ 2 teaspoon olive oil

DIRECTIONS:

- ➢ Sprinkle the sliced bacon with ground black pepper and dried rosemary.
- ➢ Wrap every Mozzarella ball in the sliced bacon and secure them with toothpicks.
- ➢ Brush wrapped Mozzarella balls with oil.
- ➢ Line the baking tray with the parchment and arrange Mozzarella balls in it.
- ➢ Bake the meal for 10 minutes at 365F.

NUTRITION INFORMATION: Calories: 323 Fat: 26.8 Fiber: 0.1 Carbs: 0.6 Protein: 20.6

104. COLESLAW ASIAN STYLE

Servings: 10 **Cook Time: 0 Min** **Prep Time 10 Min**

INGREDIENTS:

- ½ cup chopped fresh cilantro
- 1 ½ tbsp minced garlic
- 2 carrots, julienned
- 2 cups shredded napa cabbage
- 2 cups thinly sliced red cabbage
- 2 red bell peppers, thinly sliced
- 2 tbsp minced fresh ginger root
- 3 tbsp brown sugar
- 3 tbsp soy sauce
- 5 cups thinly sliced green cabbage
- 5 tbsp creamy peanut butter
- 6 green onions, chopped
- 6 tbsp rice wine vinegar
- 6 tbsp vegetable oil

DIRECTIONS:

- Mix thoroughly the following in a medium bowl: garlic, ginger, brown sugar
- Add soy sauce, peanut butter, oil and rice vinegar
- In a separate bowl, blend well cilantro, green onions, carrots, bell pepper
- Then Napa cabbage, red cabbage and green cabbage
- Pour in the peanut sauce above
- Toss to mix well
- Serve and enjoy.

NUTRITION INFORMATION: Calories: 193.8; Protein: 4g; Fat: 12.6g; Carbs: 16.1g

105. CUCUMBER SALAD JAPANESE STYLE

Servings: 5 **Cook Time: 0 Min** **Prep Time 10 Min**

INGREDIENTS:

- ½ tsp minced fresh ginger root
- 1 tsp salt
- 1/3 cup rice vinegar
- 2 large cucumbers, ribbon cut
- 4 tsp white sugar

DIRECTIONS:

- Mix well ginger, salt, sugar and vinegar in a small bowl
- Add ribbon cut cucumbers and mix well
- Let stand for at least one hour in the ref before serving.

NUTRITION INFORMATION: Calories: 29; Fat: .2g; Protein: .7g; Carbs: 6.1g

106. GARLIC CHICKEN BALLS

Servings: 4 **Cook Time: 10 Min** **Prep Time 15 Min**

INGREDIENTS:

- ✓ 2 cups ground chicken
- ✓ 1 teaspoon minced garlic
- ✓ 1 teaspoon dried dill
- ✓ 1/3 carrot, grated
- ✓ 1 egg, beaten
- ✓ 1 tablespoon olive oil
- ✓ 1/4 cup coconut flakes
- ✓ 1/2 teaspoon salt

DIRECTIONS:

- ➢ In the mixing bowl mix up together ground chicken, minced garlic, dried dill, carrot, egg, and salt.
- ➢ Stir the chicken mixture with the help of the fingertips until homogenous.
- ➢ Then make medium balls from the mixture.
- ➢ Coat every chicken ball in coconut flakes.
- ➢ Heat up olive oil in the skillet.
- ➢ Add chicken balls and cook them for 3 minutes from each side
- ➢ The cooked chicken balls will have a golden-brown color.

NUTRITION INFORMATION: Calories: 200 Fat: 11.5 Fiber: 0.6 Carbs: 1.7 Protein: 21.9

107. GARLICKY SAUTÉED ZUCCHINI WITH MINT

Servings: 4 **Cook Time: 10 Min** **Prep Time 5 Min**

INGREDIENTS:

- ✓ 3 large green zucchinis
- ✓ 3 tablespoons extra-virgin olive oil
- ✓ 1 large onion, chopped
- ✓ 3 cloves garlic, minced
- ✓ 1 teaspoon dried mint

DIRECTIONS:

- ➢ Cut the zucchini into ½-inch cubes.
- ➢ Using huge skillet, place over medium heat
- ➢ Cook the olive oil, onions, and garlic for 3 minutes, stirring constantly.
- ➢ Add the zucchini and salt to the skillet
- ➢ Toss to combine with the onions and garlic, cooking for 5 minutes.
- ➢ Add the mint to the skillet, tossing to combine
- ➢ Cook for another 2 minutes. Serve warm.

NUTRITION INFORMATION: Calories: 147 Protein: 4g Carbohydrates: 12g

108. STEWED OKRA

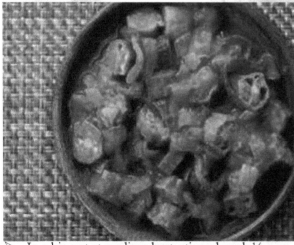

Servings: 4 **Cook Time: 25Min**
Prep Time 5 Min

INGREDIENTS:

- ✓ 3 cloves garlic, finely chopped
- ✓ 1 pound fresh or frozen okra, cleaned
- ✓ 1 (15-ounce) can plain tomato sauce
- ✓ 2 cups water
- ✓ ½ cup fresh cilantro, finely chopped

DIRECTIONS:

- ➢ Stir in the okra and cook for 3 minutes.
- ➢ Add the tomato sauce, water, cilantro, and black pepper
- ➢ Stir, cover, and let cook for 15 minutes, stirring occasionally.
- ➢ Serve warm.
- ➢ In a big pot at medium heat, stir and cook ¼ cup of olive oil, 1 onion, garlic, and salt for 1 minute.

NUTRITION INFORMATION: Calories: 201 Protein: 4g Carbohydrates: 18g

109. SWEET VEGGIE-STUFFED PEPPERS

Servings: 6　　　　**Cook Time: 30 Min**　　　　**Prep Time 20 Min**

INGREDIENTS:

- ✓ 6 large bell peppers, different colors
- ✓ 3 cloves garlic, minced
- ✓ 1 carrot, chopped
- ✓ (16-ounce) can garbanzo beans
- ✓ 3 cups cooked rice

DIRECTIONS:

- ➢ Preheat the oven to 350°F.
- ➢ Make sure to choose peppers that can stand upright
- ➢ Cut off the pepper cap and remove the seeds, reserving the cap for later
- ➢ Stand the peppers in a baking dish.
- ➢ In a skillet over medium heat, cook up olive oil, 1 onion, garlic, and carrots for 3 minutes.
- ➢ Stir in the garbanzo beans. Cook for another 3 minutes.
- ➢ Remove the pan from the heat
- ➢ Spoon the cooked ingredients to a large bowl.
- ➢ Add the rice, salt, and pepper; toss to combine.
- ➢ Stuff each pepper to the top and then put the pepper caps back on
- ➢ Cover the baking dish with aluminum foil and bake for 25 minutes.
- ➢ Remove the foil and bake for another 5 minutes.
- ➢ Serve warm.

NUTRITION INFORMATION: Calories: 301 Protein: 8g Carbohydrates: 50g

110. VEGETABLE-STUFFED GRAPE LEAVES

Servings: 7　　　　**Cook Time: 45 Min**　　　　**Prep Time 50 Min**

INGREDIENTS:

- ✓ 1 cups white rice, rinsed
- ✓ 2 large tomatoes, finely diced
- ✓ 1 (16-ounce) jar grape leaves
- ✓ 1 cup lemon juice
- ✓ 4 to 6 cups water

DIRECTIONS:

- ➢ Incorporate rice, tomatoes, 1 onion, 1 green onion, 1 cup of parsley, 3 garlic cloves, salt, and black pepper.
- ➢ Drain and rinse the grape leaves.
- ➢ Prepare a large pot by placing a layer of grape leaves on the bottom
- ➢ Lay each leaf flat and trim off any stems.
- ➢ Place 2 tablespoons of the rice mixture at the base of each leaf
- ➢ Fold over the sides, then roll as tight as possible
- ➢ Place the rolled grape leaves in the pot, lining up each rolled grape leaf
- ➢ Continue to layer in the rolled grape leaves.
- ➢ Gently pour the lemon juice and olive oil over the grape leaves
- ➢ Add enough water to just cover the grape leaves by 1 inch.
- ➢ Lay a heavy plate that is smaller
- ➢ Than the opening of the pot upside down over the grape leaves
- ➢ Cover the pot and cook the leaves over medium-low heat for 45 minutes
- ➢ Let stand for 20 minutes before serving.
- ➢ Serve warm or cold.

NUTRITION INFORMATION: Calories: 532 Protein: 12g Carbohydrates: 80g

111. GRILLED EGGPLANT ROLLS

Servings: 5 **Cook Time: 10 Min** **Prep Time 30 Min**

INGREDIENTS:
- ✓ 2 large eggplants
- ✓ 4 ounces goat cheese
- ✓ 1 cup ricotta
- ✓ ¼ cup fresh basil, finely chopped

DIRECTIONS:
- ➢ Slice the tops of the eggplants off and cut the eggplants lengthwise into ¼-inch-thick slices
- ➢ Sprinkle the slices with the salt and place the eggplant in a colander for 15 to 20 minutes
- ➢ The salt will draw out excess water from the eggplant.
- ➢ In a large bowl, combine the goat cheese, ricotta, basil, and pepper
- ➢ Preheat a grill, grill pan, or lightly oiled skillet on medium heat
- ➢ Pat the eggplant slices dry using paper towel and lightly spray with olive oil spray
- ➢ Place the eggplant on the grill, grill pan, or skillet and cook for 3 minutes on each side.
- ➢ Remove the eggplant from the heat and let cool for 5 minutes.
- ➢ To roll, lay one eggplant slice flat
- ➢ Place a tablespoon of the cheese mixture at the base of the slice, and roll up
- ➢ Serve immediately or chill until serving.

NUTRITION INFORMATION: Calories: 255 Protein: 15g Carbohydrates: 19g

112. CRISPY ZUCCHINI FRITTERS

Servings: 6 **Cook Time: 20 Min** **Prep Time 15 Min**

INGREDIENTS:
- ✓ 2 large green zucchinis
- ✓ 1 cup flour
- ✓ 1 large egg, beaten
- ✓ ½ cup water
- ✓ 1 teaspoon baking powder

DIRECTIONS:
- ➢ Grate the zucchini into a large bowl.
- ➢ Add the 2 tbsps. of parsley, 3 garlic cloves, salt, flour, egg, water
- ➢ Then baking powder to the bowl and stir to combine.
- ➢ In a large pot or fryer over medium heat, heat oil to 365°F.
- ➢ Drop the fritter batter into 3 cups of vegetable oil
- ➢ Turn the fritters over using a slotted spoon and fry
- ➢ (Until they are golden brown, about 2 to 3 minutes)
- ➢ Strain fritters from the oil
- ➢ Place on a plate lined with paper towels.
- ➢ Serve warm with Creamy Tzatziki or Creamy Traditional Hummus as a dip.

NUTRITION INFORMATION: Calories: 446 Protein: 5g Carbohydrates: 19g

113. CHEESY SPINACH PIES

Servings: 5 **Cook Time: 40 Min** **Prep Time 20 Min**

INGREDIENTS:

- ✓ 1 tablespoons extra-virgin olive oil
- ✓ 2 (1-pound) bags of baby spinach, washed
- ✓ 1 cup feta cheese
- ✓ 1 large egg, beaten
- ✓ Puff pastry sheets

DIRECTIONS:

- ➢ Preheat the oven to 375°F.
- ➢ In a frying pan on medium heat, put the olive oil, 1 onion, and 2 garlic cloves for 3 minutes.
- ➢ Add the spinach to the skillet one bag at a time, letting it wilt in between each bag
- ➢ Toss using tongs. Cook for 4 minutes
- ➢ Once the spinach is cooked, drain any excess liquid from the pan.
- ➢ Mix feta cheese, egg, and cooked spinach.
- ➢ Lay the puff pastry flat on a counter
- ➢ Cut the pastry into 3-inch squares.
- ➢ Place a tablespoon of the spinach mixture in the center of a puff-pastry square
- ➢ Fold over one corner of the square to the diagonal corner, forming a triangle
- ➢ Crimp the edges of the pie by pressing down with the tines of a fork to seal them together
- ➢ Repeat until all squares are filled.
- ➢ Situate the pies on a parchment-lined baking sheet
- ➢ Bake for 25 to 30 minutes or until golden brown
- ➢ Serve warm or at room temperature

NUTRITION INFORMATION: Calories: 503 Protein: 16g Carbohydrates: 38g

114. *SEA BASS CRUSTED WITH MOROCCAN SPICES*

Servings: 4   **Cook Time: 40 Min**   **Prep Time 15 Min**

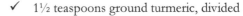

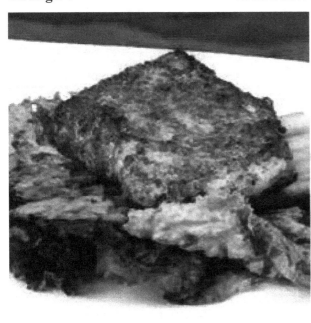

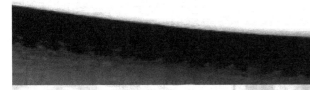

INGREDIENTS:

- ✓ 1½ teaspoons ground turmeric, divided
- ✓ ¾ teaspoon saffron
- ✓ ½ teaspoon ground cumin
- ✓ ¼ teaspoon kosher salt
- ✓ ¼ teaspoon freshly ground black pepper
- ✓ 1½ pounds (680 g) sea bass fillets, about
- ✓ ½ inch thick 8 tablespoons extra-virgin olive oil, divided
- ✓ 8 garlic cloves, divided (4 minced cloves and 4 sliced)
- ✓ 6 medium baby portobello mushrooms, chopped
- ✓ 1 large carrot, sliced on an angle
- ✓ 2 sun-dried tomatoes, thinly sliced (optional)
- ✓ 2 tablespoons tomato paste
- ✓ 1 (15-ounce / 425-g) can chickpeas, drained and rinsed
- ✓ 1½ cups low-sodium vegetable broth
- ✓ ¼ cup white wine
- ✓ 1 tablespoon ground coriander (optional)
- ✓ 1 cup sliced artichoke hearts marinated in olive oil
- ✓ ½ cup pitted Kalamata olives
- ✓ ½ lemon, juiced
- ✓ ½ lemon, cut into thin rounds
- ✓ 4 to 5 rosemary sprigs or
- ✓ 2 tablespoons dried rosemary
- ✓ Fresh cilantro, for garnish

DIRECTIONS:

- ➢ In a small mixing bowl, combine 1 teaspoon turmeric and the saffron and cumin
- ➢ Season with salt and pepper. Season both sides of the fish with the spice mixture
- ➢ Add 3 tablespoons of olive oil
- ➢ Work the fish to make sure it's well coated with the spices and the olive oil.
- ➢ In a large sauté pan or skillet, heat 2 tablespoons of olive oil over medium heat until shimmering but not smoking
- ➢ Sear the top side of the sea bass for about 1 minute, or until golden
- ➢ Remove and set aside.
- ➢ In the same skillet, add the minced garlic and cook very briefly, tossing regularly, until fragrant
- ➢ Add the mushrooms, carrot, sun-dried tomatoes (if using), and tomato paste
- ➢ Cook for 3 to 4 minutes over medium heat, tossing frequently, until fragrant
- ➢ Add the chickpeas, broth, wine, coriander (if using), and the sliced garlic
- ➢ Stir in the remaining ½ teaspoon ground turmeric
- ➢ Raise the heat, if needed, and bring to a boil, then lower heat to simmer
- ➢ Cover part of the way and let the sauce simmer for about 20 minutes, until thickened.
- ➢ Carefully add the seared fish to the skillet
- ➢ Ladle a bit of the sauce on top of the fish
- ➢ Add the artichokes, olives, lemon juice and slices, and rosemary sprigs
- ➢ Cook another 10 minutes or until the fish is fully cooked and flaky
- ➢ Garnish with fresh cilantro.

NUTRITION INFORMATION: Calories: 696 fat: 41g protein: 48g carbs: 37g fiber: 9g sodium: 810mg

115. *INSTANT POT BLACK EYED PEAS*

Servings: 4   **Cook Time: 25 Min**   **Prep Time 6 Min**

INGREDIENTS:

- ✓ 2 cups black-eyed peas (dried)
- ✓ 1 cup parsley, dill
- ✓ 2 slices oranges, 2 tbsp. tomato paste

- ✓ 4 green onions
- ✓ 2 carrots, bay leaves

DIRECTIONS:

- ➤ Clean the dill thoroughly with water removing stones.
- ➤ Add all the ingredients in the instant pot and stir well to combine.

- ➤ Lid the instant pot and set the vent to sealing.
- ➤ Set time for twenty-five minutes
- ➤ When the time has elapsed release pressure naturally.

NUTRITION INFORMATION: Calories: 506 Protein: 14g Carbohydrates: 33g

116. *GREEN BEANS AND POTATOES IN OLIVE OIL*

Servings: 4   **Cook Time: 17 Min**   **Prep Time 12 Min**

INGREDIENTS:

- ✓ 15 oz. tomatoes (diced)
- ✓ 2 potatoes
- ✓ 1 lb. green beans (fresh)
- ✓ 1 bunch dill, parsley, zucchini
- ✓ 1 tbsp. dried oregano

DIRECTIONS:

- ➤ Turn on the sauté function on your instant pot.
- ➤ Pour tomatoes, a cup of water and olive oil
- ➤ Add the rest of the ingredients and stir through.
- ➤ Lid the instant pot and set the valve to seal

- ➤ Set time for fifteen minutes.
- ➤ When the time has elapsed release pressure
- ➤ Remove the Fasolakia from the instant pot
- ➤ Serve and enjoy.

NUTRITION INFORMATION: Calories: 510 Protein: 20g Carbohydrates: 28g

117. *BEEF STRIPS WITH LETTUCE SALAD*

Servings: 5   **Cook Time: 12 Min**   **Prep Time 10 Min**

INGREDIENTS:

- ✓ 1 cup lettuce
- ✓ 10 oz. beef brisket
- ✓ 2 tablespoon sesame oil
- ✓ 1 tablespoon sunflower seeds
- ✓ 1 cucumber

- ✓ 1 teaspoon ground black pepper
- ✓ 1 teaspoon paprika
- ✓ 1 teaspoon Italian spices 2 teaspoon butter
- ✓ 1 teaspoon dried dill
- ✓ 2 tablespoon coconut milk

DIRECTIONS:

- ➤ Cut the beef brisket into strips.
- ➤ Sprinkle the beef strips with the ground black pepper, paprika, and dried dill.
- ➤ Preheat the air fryer to 365 F.
- ➤ Put the butter in the air fryer basket tray and melt it.
- ➤ Then add the beef strips and cook them for 6 minutes on each side.
- ➤ Meanwhile, tear the lettuce and toss it in a big salad bowl.
- ➤ Crush the sunflower seeds and sprinkle over the lettuce.
- ➤ Chop the cucumber into the small cubes and add to the salad bowl.

- ➤ Then combine the sesame oil and Italian spices together. Stir the oil.
- ➤ Combine the lettuce mixture with the coconut milk and stir it using 2 wooden spatulas.
- ➤ When the meat is cooked – let it chill to room temperature.
- ➤ Add the beef strips to the salad bowl.
- ➤ Stir it gently and sprinkle the salad with the sesame oil dressing.
- ➤ Serve the dish immediately.

NUTRITION INFORMATION: Calories: 199 Fat: 12.4g Carbs: 3.9g Protein: 18.1g

118. NUTRITIOUS VEGAN CABBAGE

Servings: 6   **Cook Time: 15 Min**   **Prep Time 35 Min**

INGREDIENTS:

- ✓ 3 cups green cabbage
- ✓ 1 can tomatoes, onion
- ✓ Cups vegetable broth
- ✓ 3 stalks celery, carrots
- ✓ 2 tbsp. vinegar, sage

DIRECTIONS:

- ➤ Mix 1 tbsp. of lemon juice. 2 garlic cloves and the rest of ingredients in the instant pot and
- ➤ Lid and set time for fifteen minutes on high pressure.
- ➤ Release pressure naturally then remove the lid
- ➤ Remove the soup from the instant pot.
- ➤ Serve and enjoy.

NUTRITION INFORMATION: Calories: 67 Fat: 0.4g Fiber: 3.8g

119. INSTANT POT HORTA AND POTATOES

Servings: 4   **Cook Time: 17 Min**   **Prep Time 12 Min**

INGREDIENTS:

- ✓ 2 heads of washed and chopped greens (spinach, Dandelion, kale, mustard green, Swiss chard)
- ✓ 6 potatoes (washed and cut in pieces)
- ✓ 1 cup virgin olive oil
- ✓ 1 lemon juice (reserve slices for serving)
- ✓ 10 garlic cloves (chopped)

DIRECTIONS:

- ➤ Position all the ingredients in the instant pot and lid setting the vent to sealing.
- ➤ Set time for fifteen minutes
- ➤ When time is done release pressure.
- ➤ Let the potatoes rest for some time
- ➤ Serve and enjoy with lemon slices.

NUTRITION INFORMATION: Calories: 499 Protein: 18g Carbohydrates: 41g

120. INSTANT POT JACKFRUIT CURRY

Servings: 2   **Cook Time: 16 Min**   **Prep Time 1 H**

INGREDIENTS:

- ✓ 1 tbsp. oil
- ✓ Cumin seeds, Mustard seeds
- ✓ 2 tomatoes (purred)
- ✓ 20 oz. can green jackfruit (drained and rinsed)
- ✓ 1 tbsp. coriander powder, turmeric.

DIRECTIONS:

- ➤ Turn the instant pot to sauté mode
- ➤ Add cumin plus mustard seeds, then allow them to sizzle.
- ➤ Add other ingredients, and a cup of water then lid the instant pot
- ➤ Set time for seven minutes on high pressure.
- ➤ When the time has elapsed release pressure naturally
- ➤ Shred the jackfruit and serve.

NUTRITION INFORMATION: Calories: 369 Fat: 3g Fiber: 6g

121. BEAN FRITTATA WITH SWEET POTATOES

Servings: 4   **Cook Time: 20 Min**   **Prep Time 25 Min**

INGREDIENTS:

- ✓ 4 eggs, whisked
- ✓ 1 red onion, chopped
- ✓ 2 tbsp olive oil
- ✓ 2 sweet potatoes, boiled and chopped
- ✓ ¾ cup ham, chopped
- ✓ ½ cup white beans, cooked
- ✓ 2 tbsp Greek yogurt Salt and black pepper to taste
- ✓ ½ cup cherry tomatoes, halved
- ✓ ¾ cup cheddar cheese, grated

DIRECTIONS:

- ➤ Warm the olive oil in a skillet over medium heat and sauté onion for 2 minutes
- ➤ Stir in sweet potatoes, ham, beans, yogurt, salt, pepper, and tomatoes
- ➤ Cook for another 3 minutes
- ➤ Pour in eggs and cheese, lock the lid
- ➤ Cook for an additional 10 minutes
- ➤ Cut before serving.

NUTRITION INFORMATION: Calories 280, Fat 18g, Carbs 9g, Protein 12g

122. SHRIMP WITH GARLIC AND MUSHROOMS

Servings: 4   **Cook Time: 15 Min**   **Prep Time 10 Min**

INGREDIENTS:

- ✓ 1 pound (454 g) peeled and deveined fresh shrimp
- ✓ 1 teaspoon salt
- ✓ 1 cup extra-virgin olive oil
- ✓ 8 large garlic cloves, thinly sliced
- ✓ 4 ounces (113 g) sliced mushrooms (shiitake, baby bella, or button)
- ✓ ½ teaspoon red pepper flakes
- ✓ ¼ cup chopped fresh flat-leaf Italian parsley
- ✓ Zucchini noodles or riced cauliflower, for serving

DIRECTIONS:

- ➤ Rinse the shrimp and pat dry
- ➤ Place in a small bowl and sprinkle with the salt.
- ➤ In a large rimmed, thick skillet, heat the olive oil over medium-low heat
- ➤ Add the garlic and heat until very fragrant, 3 to 4 minutes
- ➤ Reduce the heat if the garlic starts to burn.
- ➤ Add the mushrooms and sauté for 5 minutes, until softened
- ➤ Then the shrimp and red pepper flakes and sauté
- ➤ (Until the shrimp begins to turn pink, another 3 to 4 minutes)
- ➤ Remove from the heat and stir in the parsley
- ➤ Serve over zucchini noodles or riced cauliflower.

NUTRITION INFORMATION: Calories: 620 fat: 56g protein: 24g carbs: 4g fiber: 0g sodium: 736mg

123. NACHOS

Servings: 4   **Cook Time: 10 Min**   **Prep Time 5 Min**

INGREDIENTS:

- ✓ 4-ounce restaurant-style corn tortilla chips
- ✓ 1 medium green onion, thinly sliced (about 1 tbsp.)
- ✓ 1 (4 ounces) package finely crumbled feta cheese
- ✓ 1 finely chopped and drained plum tomato
- ✓ 2 tbsp Sun-dried tomatoes in oil, finely chopped
- ✓ 2 tbsp Kalamata olives

DIRECTIONS:

- ➤ Mix an onion, plum tomato, oil, sun-dried tomatoes, and olives in a small bowl.
- ➤ Arrange the tortillas chips on a microwavable plate in a single layer topped evenly with cheese
- ➤ (Microwave on high for one minute)
- ➤ Rotate the plate half turn and continue microwaving until the cheese is bubbly
- ➤ Spread the tomato mixture over the chips and cheese and enjoy.

NUTRITION INFORMATION: Calories: 140 Carbs: 19g Fat: 7g Protein: 2g

124. STUFFED CELERY

Servings: 3 **Cook Time: 20 Min** **Prep Time 15 Min**

INGREDIENTS:

- ✓ Olive oil
- ✓ 1 clove garlic, minced 2 tbsp Pine nuts
- ✓ 2 tbsp dry-roasted sunflower seeds
- ✓ ¼ cup Italian cheese blend, shredded
- ✓ 8 stalks celery leaves
- ✓ 1 (8-ounce) fat-free cream cheese
- ✓ Cooking spray

DIRECTIONS:

- ➤ Sauté garlic and pine nuts over a medium setting for the heat
- ➤ (Until the nuts are golden brown)
- ➤ Cut off the wide base and tops from celery.
- ➤ Remove two thin strips from the round side of the celery to create a flat surface.
- ➤ Mix Italian cheese and cream cheese in a bowl
- ➤ Spread into cut celery stalks.
- ➤ Sprinkle half of the celery pieces with sunflower seeds and a half with the pine nut mixture
- ➤ Cover mixture and let stand for at least 4 hours before eating.

NUTRITION INFORMATION: Calories: 64 Carbs: 2g Fat: 6g Protein: 1g

125. CLASSIC ESCABECHE

Servings: 4 **Cook Time: 20 Min** **Prep Time 10 Min**

INGREDIENTS:

- ✓ 1 pound (454 g) wild-caught Spanish mackerel fillets, cut into four pieces
- ✓ 1 teaspoon salt
- ✓ ½ teaspoon freshly ground black pepper
- ✓ 8 tablespoons extra-virgin olive oil, divided
- ✓ 1 bunch asparagus, trimmed and cut into 2-inch pieces
- ✓ 1 (13¾-ounce / 390-g) can artichoke hearts, drained and quartered
- ✓ 4 large garlic cloves, peeled and crushed
- ✓ 2 bay leaves
- ✓ ¼ cup red wine vinegar
- ✓ ½ teaspoon smoked paprika

DIRECTIONS:

- ➤ Sprinkle the fillets with salt and pepper and let sit at room temperature for 5 minutes.
- ➤ In a large skillet, heat 2 tablespoons olive oil over medium-high heat
- ➤ Add the fish, skin-side up, and cook 5 minutes
- ➤ Flip and cook 5 minutes on the other side, until browned and cooked through
- ➤ Transfer to a serving dish, pour the cooking oil over the fish, and cover to keep warm.
- ➤ Heat the remaining 6 tablespoons olive oil in the same skillet over medium heat
- ➤ Add the asparagus, artichokes, garlic, and bay
- ➤ Leaves and sauté until the vegetables are tender, 6 to 8 minutes.
- ➤ Use slotted spoon
- ➤ Top the fish with the cooked vegetables, reserving the oil in the skillet
- ➤ Then the vinegar and paprika to the oil and whisk to combine well
- ➤ Pour the vinaigrette over the fish and vegetables
- ➤ Let sit at room temperature for at least 15 minutes
- ➤ (Or marinate in the refrigerator up to 24 hours for a deeper flavor)
- ➤ Remove the bay leaf before serving.

NUTRITION INFORMATION: Calories: 578 fat: 50g protein: 26g carbs: 13g fiber: 5g sodium: 946mg

126. OLIVE OIL-POACHED TUNA

Servings: 4   **Cook Time: 45 Min**   **Prep Time 15 Min**

INGREDIENTS:

- ✓ 1 cup extra-virgin olive oil, plus more if needed
- ✓ 4 (3- to 4-inch) sprigs fresh rosemary
- ✓ 8 (3- to 4-inch) sprigs fresh thyme
- ✓ 2 large garlic cloves, thinly sliced
- ✓ 2 (2-inch) strips lemon zest
- ✓ 1 teaspoon salt
- ✓ ½ teaspoon freshly ground black pepper
- ✓ 1 pound (454 g) fresh tuna steaks (about 1 inch thick)

DIRECTIONS:

- ➤ Select a thick pot just large enough to fit the tuna in a single layer on the bottom
- ➤ The larger the pot, the more olive oil you will need to use
- ➤ Combine the olive oil, rosemary, thyme, garlic, lemon zest, salt, and pepper over medium-low heat
- ➤ Cook until warm and fragrant, 20 to 25 minutes, lowering the heat if it begins to smoke.
- ➤ Remove from the heat and allow to cool for 25 to 30 minutes, until warm but not hot.
- ➤ Add the tuna to the bottom of the pan, adding additional oil if needed
- ➤ So that tuna is fully submerged, and return to medium-low heat
- ➤ Cook for 5 to 10 minutes
- ➤ (Or until the oil heats back up and is warm and fragrant but not smoking)
- ➤ Lower the heat if it gets too hot.
- ➤ Remove the pot from the heat and let the tuna cook in warm oil 4 to 5 minutes, to your desired level of doneness
- ➤ For a tuna that is rare in the center, cook for 2 to 3 minutes.
- ➤ Remove from the oil and serve warm, drizzling 2 to 3 tablespoons seasoned oil over the tuna.
- ➤ To store for later use, remove the tuna from the oil
- ➤ Place in a container with a lid
- ➤ Allow tuna and oil to cool separately. When both have cooled
- ➤ Remove the herb stems with a slotted spoon and pour the cooking oil over the tuna
- ➤ Cover and store in the refrigerator for up to 1 week
- ➤ Bring to room temperature to allow the oil to liquify before serving.

NUTRITION INFORMATION: Calories: 363 fat: 28g protein: 27g carbs: 1g fiber: 0g sodium: 624mg

127. ITALIAN SPINACH & RICE SALAD

Servings: 2   **Cook Time: 45 Min**   **Prep Time 30 Min**

INGREDIENTS:

- ✓ 1 tbsp olive oil Salt and black pepper to taste
- ✓ ½ cup baby spinach ½ cup green peas, blanched
- ✓ 1 garlic clove, minced ½ cup white rice, rinsed
- ✓ ½ cup cherry tomatoes, halved
- ✓ 1 tbsp parsley, chopped
- ✓ 2 tbsp Italian salad dressing

DIRECTIONS:

- ➤ Bring a large pot of salted water to a boil over medium heat
- ➤ Pour in the rice, cover, and simmer on a low heat for 15-18 minutes
- ➤ (Or until until the rice is al dente)
- ➤ Drain and let cool into a salad bowl
- ➤ In a bowl, whisk the olive oil, garlic, salt, and black pepper
- ➤ Toss the green peas, baby spinach, and rice together
- ➤ Pour the dressing all over and gently stir to combine
- ➤ Decorate with cherry tomatoes and parsley and serve. Enjoy!

NUTRITION INFORMATION: Calories 160, Fat 14g, Carbs 9g, Protein 4g

128. FRUITY ASPARAGUS-QUINOA SALAD

Servings: 8   **Cook Time: 25 Min**   **Prep Time 25 Min**

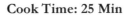

INGREDIENTS:

- ✓ ¼ cup chopped pecans, toasted
- ✓ ½ cup finely chopped white onion
- ✓ ½ jalapeno pepper, diced
- ✓ ½ lb. asparagus, sliced to
- ✓ 2-inch lengths, steamed and chilled
- ✓ ½ tsp kosher salt
- ✓ 1 cup fresh orange sections
- ✓ 1 cup uncooked quinoa
- ✓ 1 tsp olive oil
- ✓ 2 cups water
- ✓ 2 tbsp minced red onion
- ✓ 5 dates, pitted and chopped

- ✓ 2 tbsp chopped fresh mint
- ✓ 2 tbsp fresh lemon juice Mint sprigs(optional)

DRESSING INGREDIENTS:
- ✓ ¼ tsp ground black pepper
- ✓ ¼ tsp kosher salt 1 garlic clove, minced
- ✓ 1 tbsp olive oil

DIRECTIONS:
- ➢ Wash and rub with your hands the quinoa in a bowl at least three times, discarding water each and every time
- ➢ On medium high fire, place a large nonstick fry pan and heat 1 tsp olive oil
- ➢ For two minutes, sauté onions before adding quinoa and sautéing for another five minutes
- ➢ Add ½ tsp salt and 2 cups water and bring to a boil

- ➢ Lower fire to a simmer, cover and cook for 15 minutes
- ➢ Turn off fire and let stand until water is absorbed
- ➢ Then pepper asparagus, dates, pecans and orange sections into a salad bowl
- ➢ Join also cooked quinoa, toss to mix well
- ➢ In a small bowl, whisk mint, garlic, black pepper, salt, olive oil and lemon juice to create the dressing
- ➢ Pour dressing over salad, serve and enjoy.

NUTRITION INFORMATION: Calories: 173; Fat: 6.3g; Protein: 4.3g; Carbohydrates: 24.7g

129. ZA'ATAR SALMON WITH CUCUMBER SALAD

Servings: 4   **Cook Time: 25 Min**   **Prep Time 5 Min**

INGREDIENTS:
SALAD
- ✓ 4 cups sliced cucumber
- ✓ 1 pint cherry tomatoes, halved
- ✓ 1/4 cup chopped fresh dill
SALMON:
- ✓ 11/2 pounds (680 g) skinless salmon
- ✓ 1 tablespoon Za'atar

- ✓ 1/4 cup cider vinegar
- ✓ 1/4 teaspoon salt
- ✓ 1/4 teaspoon black pepper

- ✓ 4 lemon wedges

DIRECTIONS:
- ➢ Preheat the oven to 350°F (180°C). Line a baking sheet with aluminum foil.
- ➢ Toss all the salad ingredients in a bowl until combined. Set aside.
- ➢ Season the salmon with Za'atar on both sides

- ➢ Place on the prepared baking sheet. Roast in the preheated oven for about 25 minutes
- ➢ (Or until the internal temperature registers 145°F (63°C))
- ➢ Serve the salmon with the salad and lemon wedges.

NUTRITION INFORMATION: 1 Lean 3 Greens 3 Condiments

130. GARDEN SALAD WITH ORANGES AND OLIVES

Servings: 4   **Cook Time: 15 Min**   **Prep Time 15 Min**

INGREDIENTS:

- ½ cup red wine vinegar
- 1 tbsp extra virgin olive oil
- 1 tbsp finely chopped celery
- 1 tbsp finely chopped red onion
- 16 large ripe black olives
- 2 garlic cloves

- 2 navel oranges, peeled and segmented
- 4 boneless, skinless chicken breasts
- 4-oz each 4 garlic cloves, minced
- 8 cups leaf lettuce, washed and dried
- Cracked black pepper to taste

DIRECTIONS:

- Prepare the dressing by mixing pepper, celery, onion, olive oil, garlic and vinegar in a small bowl
- Whisk well to combine. Lightly grease grate and preheat grill to high
- Rub chicken with the garlic cloves and discard garlic
- Grill chicken for 5 minutes per side or until cooked through

- Remove from grill and let it stand for 5 minutes before cutting into ½-inch strips
- In 4 serving plates, evenly arrange two cups lettuce, ¼ of the sliced oranges and 4 olives per plate
- Top each plate with ¼ serving of grilled chicken, evenly drizzle with dressing
- Serve and enjoy.

NUTRITION INFORMATION: Calories: 259.8; Protein: 48.9g; Carbs: 12.9g; Fat: 1.4g

131. CAULIFLOWER GRITS, SHRIMP AND CREAMY

Servings: 2   **Cook Time: 15 Min**   **Prep Time 10 Min**

INGREDIENTS:

- 1 pound (454 g) raw, peeled and deveined shrimp
- 1/2 tablespoon Cajun seasoning
- Cooking spray
- 1/4 cup chicken broth
- 1 tablespoon lemon juice
- 1 tablespoon butter

- 2 1/2 cups finely riced cauliflower
- 1/2 cup unsweetened almond or cashew milk
- 1/4 teaspoon salt
- 1/3 cup reduced-fat shredded Cheddar cheese
- 2 tablespoons sour cream
- 1/4 cup thinly sliced scallions

DIRECTIONS:

- Add the shrimp and Cajun seasoning into a large, resealable plastic bag
- Seal the bag and toss to coat well.
- Grease a skillet with cooking spray and heat over medium heat.
- Then the shrimp and cook each side for about 2 to 3 minutes
- Join also chicken broth and lemon juice, scraping any bits off of the bottom of the pan
- Let simmer for 1 minute. Remove from the heat and set aside

- In a separate skillet, melt the butter over medium heat.
- Add the riced cauliflower and cook for 5 minutes
- Then milk and salt and cook for an additional 5 minutes.
- Remove from heat and stir in sour cream and cheese until melted.
- Serve the shrimp over cauliflower grits and sprinkle with the scallions.

NUTRITION INFORMATION: 1 Leanest 3 Greens 2 Healthy Fats 3 Condiments

132. CHICKEN WITH SWIMMING RAMA

Servings: 4   **Cook Time: 10 Min**   **Prep Time 10 Min**

INGREDIENTS:

- ✓ 2 pounds chicken breast tenders or chicken breasts cut into
- ✓ 1-2 inch strips
- ✓ 8 wooden or metal kebab skewers
- ✓ 2 teaspoons turmeric
- ✓ 1 cup Coconut Milk, divided
- ✓ 1/4 cup powdered peanut butter
- ✓ 1 tablespoon soy sauce
- ✓ 1 teaspoon grated fresh ginger
- ✓ 1 packet stevia or other non-calorie sweetener
- ✓ 2 1/2 cups of your favorite low-carbohydrate stir-fry vegetables cut into bite size pieces
- ✓ (Use broccoli, cabbage, radishes, mushrooms, and peppers)

DIRECTIONS:

- ➢ Combine 1/4 cup of coconut milk and turmeric and pour over chicken
- ➢ Allow to marinate 4 hours or overnight.
- ➢ If using wooden skewers, allow to soak in water while chicken is marinating.
- ➢ Pat dry chicken. Divide chicken between skewers and set aside
- ➢ In a saucepan over medium heat combine remaining coconut milk, Peanut Butter, soy sauce and sweetener
- ➢ Stir until warmed through.
- ➢ Heat grill to high heat and grill chicken skewers 3 minutes on each side.
- ➢ Meanwhile, steam or water-sauté vegetables.
- ➢ Divide vegetables among four plates
- ➢ Top each with 2 chicken skewers and pour peanut sauce over the top.

NUTRITION INFORMATION: 325 calories, 7 grams of carbohydrates, 7 grams of fat, and 55

133. DAIKON NOODLE SALAD

Servings: 4   **Cook Time: 0 Min**   **Prep Time 10 Min**

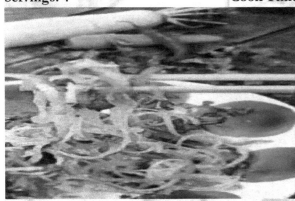

INGREDIENTS:

- ✓ 4 cups daikon radish, julienned or spiralized (see Basics: Specialized Tools)
- ✓ 1 teaspoon hot chili sauce
- ✓ 2 tablespoons lime

DIRECTIONS:

- ➢ Toss all ingredients together and chill

NUTRITION INFORMATION: 331 calories, 7 grams of carbohydrates, 4 grams of fat, and 66 grams of protein.

134. MASALA CHICKEN

Servings: 4   **Cook Time: 40 Min**   **Prep Time 10 Min**

INGREDIENTS:

- ✓ 1 1/2 pounds boneless skinless chicken breast, cut in large chunks
- ✓ 2 tablespoons butter
- ✓ 2 teaspoons masala
- ✓ 1 tablespoon grated fresh ginger
- ✓ 2 cups canned diced tomatoes, undrained
- ✓ 1 cup chopped leeks
- ✓ 1 cup yellow squash chopped
- ✓ 2 cups cauliflower florets Salt to taste
- ✓ 1 cup plain Greek yogurt
- ✓ 1 cup chopped cilantro

DIRECTIONS:

- ➢ Spray a nonstick pan with cooking spray and heat over medium high heat.
- ➢ Add chicken and brown on all sides.
- ➢ Remove from pan and set aside.
- ➢ Reduce heat and add the butter, spices, and vegetables
- ➢ Cook, stirring occasionally
- ➢ (Until vegetables are tender and tomatoes are reduced, approximately 40 minutes)
- ➢ Remove about 1 cup of the vegetables from the pan
- ➢ Blend until smooth. Salt to taste
- ➢ Return blended vegetables and chicken to pan
- ➢ Heat until chicken is warmed through, approximately 10 minutes.
- ➢ Remove from heat and stir in 1/2 cup yogurt.
- ➢ Top with additional yogurt and cilantro.

NUTRITION INFORMATION: 311 calories, 11 grams of carbohydrates, 8 grams of fat, and 47 grams of protein.

135. FIVE-SPICE MEATBALLS

Servings: 4   **Cook Time: 30 Min**   **Prep Time 10 Min**

INGREDIENTS:

- ✓ 2 packages 99% lean ground turkey (20 oz. each)
- ✓ 1 cup ground meat mix (see Basics: Ground Meat Mix)
- ✓ 1 teaspoon ground five-spice
- ✓ 4 teaspoons Olive oil 1 clove minced garlic
- ✓ 1/2 teaspoon salt
- ✓ 4 cups baby bok choy, or bok choy cut into
- ✓ 1-inch pieces

DIRECTIONS:

- ➢ Preheat oven to 425°. Cover a baking sheet with foil.
- ➢ Combine ground turkey, ground meat mix, five-spice and salt
- ➢ Roll into one inch balls
- ➢ Place on foil-lined baking sheet.
- ➢ Bake 30 minutes or until cooked through.
- ➢ Remove pan from oven and set aside.
- ➢ Heat heavy-bottomed pan or wok to high
- ➢ Add 2 tablespoons of peanut oil and swirl around bottom of pan
- ➢ Then garlic and bok choy and stir fry quickly
- ➢ (Until bok choy is browned and heated through)
- ➢ Divide among 4 plates and top with meatballs.

NUTRITION INFORMATION: 354 Calories, 3 grams of carbohydrates, 9 grams of fat, and 67 grams of protein.

136. CHICKEN DIVAN

Servings: 4 **Cook Time: 25 Min** **Prep Time 10 Min**

INGREDIENTS:

- ✓ 18 oz. cooked turkey or chicken breast, chopped into
- ✓ 1-inch cubes
- ✓ 1 1/2 cups low-fat blend (see Basics: Low-Fat Blend)
- ✓ 1/2 tsp. chicken-flavored Better Than Bouillon
- ✓ 1/4 cup minced onion

- ✓ 2 teaspoons Dijon mustard
- ✓ 1 teaspoon dried thyme
- ✓ 1/4 cup light mayo
- ✓ 1 cup frozen broccoli florets
- ✓ 1 cup mushrooms, sliced
- ✓ 4 cups yellow summer squash
- ✓ 1/4 cup Parmesan cheese

DIRECTIONS:

- ➤ Preheat oven to 375°
- ➤ Spray large casserole with nonstick cooking spray.
- ➤ Use a vegetable peeler, peel squash into long thin strips as wide as you can
- ➤ Discard center seeds. Roll in several layers of paper towels
- ➤ Squeeze out as much of the water as possible. Set aside.

- ➤ Blend low-fat blend, mayo, bouillon concentrate, minced onion, mustard, and thyme
- ➤ Fold in chicken and vegetables.
- ➤ Pour into prepared baking dish
- ➤ Sprinkle with Parmesan
- ➤ Bake 25 minutes or until warmed through.
- ➤ Let cool 10 minutes before serving.

NUTRITION INFORMATION: 299 calories, 12 grams of carbohydrates, 8 grams of fat, and 47 grams of protein.

137. BUTTERNUT SQUASH FRIES

Servings: 2 **Cook Time: 10 Min** **Prep Time 5 Min**

INGREDIENTS:

- ✓ 1 Butternut squash
- ✓ 1 tbsp Extra virgin olive oil
- ✓ ½ tbsp Grapeseed oil
- ✓ 1/8 tsp Sea salt

DIRECTIONS:

- ➤ Remove seeds from the squash and cut into thin slices
- ➤ Coat with extra virgin olive oil and grapeseed oil
- ➤ Add a sprinkle of salt and toss to coat well.
- ➤ Arrange the squash slices onto three baking sheets
- ➤ Bake for 10 minutes until crispy.

NUTRITION INFORMATION: Calories: 40 Carbs: 10g Fat: 0g Protein: 1g

138. DRIED FIG TAPENADE

Serving: 1 **Cook Time: 0 Min** **Prep Time 5 Min**

INGREDIENTS:

- ✓ 1 cup Dried figs
- ✓ 1 cup Kalamata olives
- ✓ ½ cup Water

- ✓ 1 tbsp Chopped fresh thyme
- ✓ 1 tbsp extra virgin olive oil
- ✓ ½ tsp Balsamic vinegar

DIRECTIONS:

- ➤ Prepare figs in a food processor until well chopped
- ➤ Add water, and continue processing to form a paste.
- ➤ Then olives and pulse until well blended

- ➤ Join also. Add thyme, vinegar, and extra virgin olive oil
- ➤ Pulse until very smooth. Best served with crackers of your choice

NUTRITION INFORMATION: Calories: 249 Carbs: 64g Fat: 1g Protein: 3g

139. FIDEOS WITH SEAFOOD

Servings: 8   **Cook Time: 20 Min**   **Prep Time 15 Min**

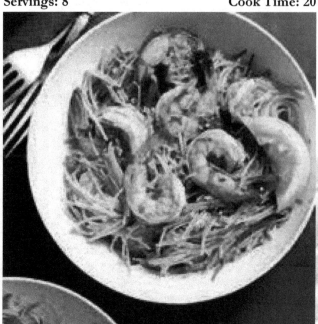

INGREDIENTS:

- ✓ 1 tablespoons extra-virgin olive oil, plus
- ✓ ½ cup, divided
- ✓ 6 cups zucchini noodles, roughly chopped (2 to 3 medium zucchini)
- ✓ 1 pound (454 g) shrimp, peeled, deveined and roughly chopped
- ✓ 6 to 8 ounces (170 to 227 g) canned chopped clams, drained
- ✓ 4 ounces (113 g) crab meat
- ✓ ½ cup crumbled goat cheese
- ✓ ½ cup crumbled feta cheese
- ✓ 1 (28-ounce / 794-g) can chopped tomatoes, with their juices
- ✓ 1 teaspoon salt
- ✓ 1 teaspoon garlic powder
- ✓ ½ teaspoon smoked paprika
- ✓ ½ cup shredded Parmesan cheese
- ✓ ¼ cup chopped fresh flat-leaf Italian parsley, for garnish

DIRECTIONS:

- ➤ Preheat the oven to 375°F (190°C).
- ➤ Pour 2 tablespoons olive oil in the bottom of a 9-by-13-inch baking dish and swirl to coat the bottom.
- ➤ In a large bowl, combine the zucchini noodles, shrimp, clams, and crab meat.
- ➤ In another bowl, combine the goat cheese, feta, and ¼ cup olive oil and stir to combine well
- ➤ Add the canned tomatoes and their juices, salt, garlic powder, and paprika and combine well.

- ➤ Then the mixture to the zucchini and seafood mixture and stir to combine.
- ➤ Pour the mixture into the prepared baking dish, spreading evenly
- ➤ Spread shredded Parmesan over top
- ➤ Drizzle with the remaining ¼ cup olive oil
- ➤ Bake until bubbly, 20 to 25 minutes
- ➤ Serve warm, garnished with chopped parsley.

NUTRITION INFORMATION: Calories: 434 fat: 31g protein: 29g carbs: 12g fiber: 3g sodium: 712mg

140. SHRIMP PESTO RICE BOWLS

Servings: 4   **Cook Time: 5 Min**   **Prep Time 5 Min**

INGREDIENTS:

- ✓ 1 pound (454 g) medium shrimp, peeled and deveined
- ✓ ¼ cup pesto sauce

- ✓ 1 lemon, sliced
- ✓ 2 cups cooked wild rice pilaf

DIRECTIONS:

- ➤ Preheat the air fryer to 360°F (182°C).
- ➤ In a medium bowl, toss the shrimp with the pesto sauce until well coated.
- ➤ Place the shrimp in a single layer in the air fryer basket

- ➤ Put the lemon slices over the shrimp and roast for 5 minutes.
- ➤ Remove the lemons and discard
- ➤ Serve a quarter of the shrimp over ½ cup wild rice with some favorite steamed vegetables.

NUTRITION INFORMATION: Calories: 249 fat: 10g protein: 20g carbs: 20g fiber: 2g sodium: 277mg

141. SALMON WITH TOMATOES AND OLIVES

Servings: 4 **Cook Time: 8 Min** **Prep Time 5 Min**

INGREDIENTS:

- ✓ 2 tablespoons olive oil
- ✓ 4 (1½-inch-thick) salmon fillets
- ✓ ½ teaspoon salt
- ✓ ¼ teaspoon cayenne
- ✓ 1 teaspoon chopped fresh dill
- ✓ 2 Roma tomatoes, diced
- ✓ ¼ cup sliced Kalamata olives 4 lemon slices

DIRECTIONS:

- ➢ Preheat the air fryer to 380°F (193°C).
- ➢ Brush the olive oil on both sides of the salmon fillets
- ➢ Then season them lightly with salt, cayenne, and dill.
- ➢ Place the fillets in a single layer in the basket of the air fryer
- ➢ Layer the tomatoes and olives over the top
- ➢ Top each fillet with a lemon slice.
- ➢ Bake for 8 minutes
- ➢ (Or until the salmon has reached an internal temperature of 145°F (63°C)).

NUTRITION INFORMATION: Calories: 241 fat: 15g protein: 23g carbs: 3g fiber: 1g sodium: 595mg

142. BAKED TROUT WITH LEMON

Servings: 4 **Cook Time: 15 Min** **Prep Time 5 Min**

INGREDIENTS:

- ✓ 4 trout fillets
- ✓ 2 tablespoons olive oil
- ✓ ½ teaspoon salt
- ✓ 1 teaspoon black pepper
- ✓ 2 garlic cloves, sliced
- ✓ 1 lemon, sliced, plus additional wedges for serving

DIRECTIONS:

- ➢ Preheat the air fryer to 380°F (193°C).
- ➢ Brush each fillet with olive oil on both sides
- ➢ Season with salt and pepper
- ➢ Place the fillets in an even layer in the air fryer basket.
- ➢ Place the sliced garlic over the tops of the trout fillets
- ➢ then top the garlic with lemon slices
- ➢ Cook for 12 to 15 minutes
- ➢ (Or until it has reached an internal temperature of 145°F (63°C))
- ➢ Serve with fresh lemon wedges.

NUTRITION INFORMATION: Calories: 231 fat: 12g protein: 29g carbs: 1g fiber: 0g sodium: 341mg

143. SPEEDY SWEET POTATO CHIPS

Servings: 4 **Cook Time: 0 Min** **Prep Time 15 Min**

INGREDIENTS:

- ✓ 1 large Sweet potato
- ✓ 1 tbsp Extra virgin olive oil
- ✓ Salt

DIRECTIONS:

- ➢ 300°F preheated oven. Slice your potato into nice, thin slices that resemble fries.
- ➢ Toss the potato slices with salt and extra virgin olive oil in a bowl
- ➢ Bake for about one hour, flipping every 15 minutes until crispy and browned

NUTRITION INFORMATION: Calories: 150 Carbs: 16g Fat: 9g Protein: 1g

144. NACHOS WITH HUMMUS (MEDITERRANEAN INSPIRED)

Servings: 4   **Cook Time: 20 Min**   **Prep Time 15 Min**

INGREDIENTS:

- ✓ 4 cups salted pita chips
- ✓ 1 (8 oz.) red pepper (roasted) Hummus
- ✓ 1 tsp Finely shredded lemon peel
- ✓ ¼ cup Chopped pitted Kalamata olives
- ✓
- ✓ ¼ cup crumbled feta cheese
- ✓ 1 plum (Roma) tomato, seeded, chopped
- ✓ ½ cup chopped cucumber
- ✓ 1 tsp Chopped fresh oregano leaves

DIRECTIONS:

- ➢ 400°F preheated oven
- ➢ Arrange the pita chips on a heatproof platter and drizzle with hummus.
- ➢ Top with olives, tomato, cucumber, cheese
- ➢ Bake until warmed through
- ➢ Sprinkle lemon zest and oregano and enjoy while it's hot.

NUTRITION INFORMATION: Calories: 130 Carbs: 18g Fat: 5g Protein: 4g

145. SEA SCALLOPS WITH WHITE BEAN PURÉE

Servings: 2   **Cook Time: 10 Min**   **Prep Time 10 Min**

INGREDIENTS:

- ✓ 4 tablespoons olive oil, divided 2 garlic cloves
- ✓ 2 teaspoons minced fresh rosemary
- ✓ 1 (15-ounce / 425-g) can white cannellini beans, drained and rinsed
- ✓ ½ cup low-sodium chicken stock
- ✓ Salt, to taste
- ✓ Freshly ground black pepper, to taste
- ✓ 6 (10 ounce / 283-g) sea scallops

DIRECTIONS:

- ➢ To make the bean purée, heat 2 tablespoons of olive oil in a saucepan over medium-high heat
- ➢ Add the garlic and sauté for 30 seconds, or just until it's fragrant
- ➢ Don't let it burn
- ➢ Then the rosemary and remove the pan from the heat.
- ➢ Add the white beans and chicken stock to the pan, return it to the heat, and stir
- ➢ Bring the beans to a boil
- ➢ Reduce the heat to low and simmer for 5 minutes.
- ➢ Transfer the beans to a blender and purée them for 30 seconds, or until they're smooth
- ➢ Taste and season with salt and pepper
- ➢ Let them sit in the blender with the lid on to keep them warm while you prepare the scallops.
- ➢ Pat the scallops dry with a paper towel
- ➢ Season them with salt and pepper.
- ➢ Heat the remaining 2 tablespoons of olive oil in a large sauté pan
- ➢ When the oil is shimmering, add the scallops, flat-side down.
- ➢ Cook the scallops for 2 minutes, or until they're golden on the bottom
- ➢ Flip them over and cook for another 1 to 2 minutes, or until opaque and slightly firm.
- ➢ To serve, divide the bean purée between two plates and top with the scallops.

NUTRITION INFORMATION: Calories: 465 fat: 28g protein: 30g carbs: 21g fiber: 7g sodium: 319mg

146. GREEN CHILI ENCHILADAS

Servings: 4   **Cook Time: 30 Min**   **Prep Time 10 Min**

INGREDIENTS:

- ✓ 14 oz. canned roasted green chilies (not jalapenos), divided
- ✓ 13 oz. canned tomatillos, drain and rinsed
- ✓ 1/2 cup leeks, chopped
- ✓ 1 cup cilantro, finely chopped, divided
- ✓ 2 cloves garlic, minced
- ✓ 12 oz. shredded low-fat cheese
- ✓ 3/4 cup 2% cottage cheese, blended until smooth
- ✓ 1/2 cup chopped mild onion
- ✓ 8 oz. turkey breast cutlets

DIRECTIONS:

- ➤ Preheat oven to 400°. Spray 9x11 baking dish with nonstick cooking spray.
- ➤ Place turkey breast cutlets between two pieces of plastic wrap
- ➤ Use a meat mallet or rolling pin, pound turkey cutlet until very thin. Set aside.
- ➤ For sauce, blend green chilies, tomatillos, leeks, 1/2 cup of cilantro, and garlic gloves until smooth. Set aside.
- ➤ For filling, combine remaining chilies, 8 oz. of shredded cheese, cottage cheese, and onion.
- ➤ Use turkey cutlet like a tortilla shell, divide filling among cutlets, roll up cutlets to form rolls
- ➤ Place seam-side down in baking dish.
- ➤ Pour sauce over cutlets, top with remaining cheese and bake 30 minutes uncovered.
- ➤ Top with remaining cilantro and serve.

NUTRITION INFORMATION: 278 Calories, 14 grams of carbohydrates, 12 grams of fat, and 25 grams of protein.

147. VEGETABLE TORTILLAS

Servings: 4   **Cook Time: 7 Min**   **Prep Time 15 Min**

INGREDIENTS:

- ✓ 2 zucchinis, cut in half, then sliced
- ✓ 1/2 inch thick 1 leek, washed and sliced
- ✓ 1 bunch scallions, cut into
- ✓ 1/2-inch pieces
- ✓ 1/4 pound (113 g) mushrooms, sliced
- ✓ 1 cup small broccoli florets
- ✓ ¾ cup water, divided
- ✓ 1 (7-0unce / 198-g) can Mexican green sauce
- ✓ 1/8 cup packed chopped fresh cilantro
- ✓ 1 tablespoon cornstarch, mixed with
- ✓ 2 tablespoons water
- ✓ 8 whole-wheat flour tortillas

DIRECTIONS:

- ➤ In a pan over medium heat, sauté the zucchinis, leek, scallions, mushrooms
- ➤ Then broccoli florets in 1/2 cup of the water for 5 minutes, or until tender-crisp.
- ➤ Stir in the remaining 1/4 cup of the water, green sauce and cilantro
- ➤ Pour in the cornstarch mixture
- ➤ Cook for 2 minutes, stirring constantly, or until thickened.
- ➤ Place a line of the vegetable mixture down the center of a tortilla
- ➤ Roll up and serve.

NUTRITION INFORMATION: Calories: 410 fat: 9.1g carbs: 73.1g protein: 11.2g fiber: 11.3g

148. SWEET POTATO AND MUSHROOM SKILLET

Servings: 4 **Cook Time: 15 Min** **Prep Time 5 Min**

INGREDIENTS:

- ✓ 1 cup low-sodium vegetable broth
- ✓ 8 ounces (227 g) mushrooms, sliced
- ✓ 4 medium sweet potatoes, cut into
- ✓ 1/2-inch dice 1 sweet onion, diced
- ✓ 1 bell pepper, diced
- ✓ 1 teaspoon garlic powder
- ✓ 1/2 teaspoon chili powder
- ✓ 1/2 teaspoon ground cumin
- ✓ 1/8 teaspoon freshly ground black pepper

DIRECTIONS:

- ➢ Heat a large skillet over medium-low heat
- ➢ Stir in all the ingredients
- ➢ Cover and cook for 10 minutes
- ➢ (Or until the sweet potatoes are easily pierced with a fork)
- ➢ Uncover and give the mixture a good stir
- ➢ Cook, uncovered, for an additional 5 minutes, stirring once halfway through.
- ➢ Serve hot.

NUTRITION INFORMATION: Calories: 159 fat: 1.2g carbs: 33.9g protein: 6.2g fiber: 5.9g

149. SAUTÉED COLLARD GREENS

Servings: 4 **Cook Time: 25 Min** **Prep Time 10 Min**

INGREDIENTS:

- ✓ 11/2 pounds (680 g) collard greens
- ✓ 1 cup low-sodium vegetable broth
- ✓ 1/2 teaspoon onion powder
- ✓ 1/2 teaspoon garlic powder
- ✓ 1/8 teaspoon freshly ground black pepper

DIRECTIONS:

- ➢ Remove the hard middle stems from the greens and roughly
- ➢ Chop the leaves into 2-inch pieces.
- ➢ In a large saucepan over medium-high heat
- ➢ Combine all the ingredients, except for the collard greens.
- ➢ Bring to a boil, then add the chopped greens
- ➢ Reduce the heat to low and cover.
- ➢ Cook for 20 minutes, stirring constantly.
- ➢ Serve warm.

NUTRITION INFORMATION: Calories: 528 fat: 55.1g carbs: 8.8g protein: 3.2g fiber: 2.3g

150. HUMMUS AND OLIVE PITA BREAD

Servings: 3 **Cook Time: 0 Min** **Prep Time 5 Min**

INGREDIENTS:

- ✓ 7 pita bread cut into 6 wedges each
- ✓ 1 (7 ounces) container plain hummus
- ✓ 1 tbsp Greek vinaigrette
- ✓ ½ cup Chopped pitted Kalamata olives

DIRECTIONS:

- ➢ Spread the hummus on a serving plate
- ➢ Mix vinaigrette and olives in a bowl and spoon over the hummus
- ➢ Enjoy with wedges of pita bread

NUTRITION INFORMATION: Calories: 225 Carbs: 40g Fat: 5g Protein: 9g

151. TAHINI VINAIGRETTE WITH CAULIFLOWER SALAD

Servings: 2   **Cook Time: 5 Min**   **Prep Time 10 Min**

INGREDIENTS:

- ✓ 1 ½ lb. of cauliflower
- ✓ ¼ cup of dried cherries
- ✓ 3 tablespoons of lemon juice
- ✓ 1 tablespoon of fresh mint, chopped
- ✓ 1 teaspoon of olive oil
- ✓ ½ cup chopped parsley

- ✓ 3 tablespoons of roasted salted pistachios, chopped
- ✓ ½ teaspoon of salt
- ✓ ¼ Cup of shallot, chopped
- ✓ 2 tablespoons of tahini

DIRECTIONS:

- ➢ Grate the cauliflower in a microwave-safe container
- ➢ Add olive oil and ¼ salt. Be sure to cover and season the cauliflower evenly
- ➢ Wrap the bowl with plastic wrap and heat it in the microwave for about 3 minutes.
- ➢ Put the rice with the cauliflower on a baking sheet

- ➢ Let cool for about 10 minutes. Add the lemon juice and the shallots.
- ➢ Let it rest to allow the cauliflower to absorb the flavor.
- ➢ Add the mixture of tahini, cherries, parsley, mint and salt
- ➢ Mix everything well. Sprinkle with roasted pistachios before serving.

NUTRITION INFORMATION: Calories:165 Fat:10g Carbohydrates:20g Protein:6g Sodium:651mg

152. MEDITERRANEAN POTATO SALAD

Servings: 2   **Cook Time: 10 Min**   **Prep Time 15 Min**

INGREDIENTS:

- ✓ 1 bunch of basil leaves, torn
- ✓ 1 garlic clove, crushed
- ✓ 1 tablespoon of olive oil
- ✓ 1 onion, sliced
- ✓ 1 teaspoon of oregano

- ✓ 100 g of roasted red pepper. Slices
- ✓ 300g potatoes, cut in half
- ✓ 1 can of cherry tomatoes
- ✓ Salt and pepper, to taste

DIRECTIONS:

Sauté the onions in a saucepan

- ➢ Add oregano and garlic. Cook everything for a minute
- ➢ Then the pepper and tomatoes. Season well
- ➢ Simmer for about 10 minutes. Put that aside.
- ➢ In a saucepan, boil the potatoes in salted water

- ➢ Cook until tender, about 15 minutes
- ➢ Drain well. Mix the potatoes with the sauce and add the basil and olives
- ➢ Finally, throw everything away before serving.

NUTRITION INFORMATION: Calories:111 Fat:9g Carbohydrates:16g Protein:3g Sodium:745mg

153. QUINOA AND PISTACHIO SALAD

Servings: 2   **Cook Time: 15 Min**   **Prep Time 10 Min**

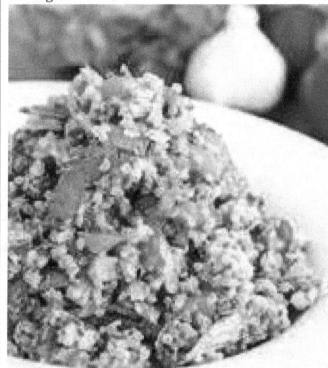

INGREDIENTS:

- ✓ ¼ teaspoon of cumin
- ✓ ½ cup of dried currants
- ✓ 1 teaspoon grated lemon zest
- ✓ 2 tablespoons of lemon juice
- ✓ ½ cup green onions, chopped
- ✓ 1 tablespoon of chopped mint
- ✓ 2 tablespoons of extra virgin olive oil
- ✓ ¼ cup chopped parsley
- ✓ ¼ teaspoon ground pepper
- ✓ 1/3 cup pistachios, chopped
- ✓ 1 ¼ cups uncooked quinoa
- ✓ 1 2/3 cup of water

DIRECTIONS:

- ➤ In a saucepan, combine 1 2/3 cups of water, raisins and quinoa.
- ➤ Cook everything until boiling then reduce the heat
- ➤ Simmer everything for about 10 minutes
- ➤ Let the quinoa become frothy. Set it aside for about 5 minutes.
- ➤ In a container, transfer the quinoa mixture
- ➤ Add the nuts, mint, onions and parsley. Mix everything.
- ➤ In separate bowl, incorporate the lemon zest, lemon juice, currants, cumin and oil
- ➤ Beat them together. Mix the dry and wet ingredients.

NUTRITION INFORMATION: Calories:248 Fat:8g Carbohydrates:35g Protein:7g Sodium:914mg

154. CUCUMBER CHICKEN SALAD WITH SPICY PEANUT DRESSING

Servings: 2   **Cook Time: 0 Min**   **Prep Time 15 Min**

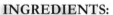

INGREDIENTS:

- ✓ 1/2 cup peanut butter
- ✓ 1 tablespoon sambal oelek (chili paste)
- ✓ 1 tablespoon low-sodium soy sauce
- ✓ 1 teaspoon grilled sesame oil
- ✓ 4 tablespoons of water, or more if necessary
- ✓ 1 cucumber with peeled and cut into thin strips
- ✓ 1 cooked chicken fillet, grated into thin strips
- ✓ 2 tablespoons chopped peanuts

DIRECTIONS:

- ➤ Combine peanut butter, soy sauce, sesame oil, sambal oelek, and water in a bowl.
- ➤ Place the cucumber slices on a dish. Garnish with grated chicken and sprinkle with sauce.
- ➤ Sprinkle the chopped peanuts.

NUTRITION INFORMATION: 720 calories 54 g fat 8.9g carbohydrates 45.9g protein 733mg sodium

155. GERMAN HOT POTATO SALAD

Servings: 12   **Cook Time: 30 Min**   **Prep Time 10 Min**

INGREDIENTS:

- ✓ 9 peeled potatoes
- ✓ 6 slices of bacon
- ✓ 1/8 teaspoon ground black pepper
- ✓ 1/2 teaspoon celery seed
- ✓ 2 tablespoons white sugar

- ✓ 2 teaspoons salt
- ✓ 3/4 cup water
- ✓ 1/3 cup distilled white vinegar
- ✓ 2 tablespoons all-purpose flour
- ✓ 3/4 cup chopped onions

DIRECTIONS:

- ➢ Boil salted water in a large pot
- ➢ Put in the potatoes and cook until soft but still firm, about 30 minutes
- ➢ Drain, let cool and cut finely.
- ➢ Over medium heat, cook bacon in a pan
- ➢ Drain, crumble and set aside. Save the cooking juices.
- ➢ Cook onions in bacon grease until golden brown.
- ➢ Combine flour, sugar, salt, celery seed, and pepper in a small bowl

- ➢ Add sautéed onions and cook
- ➢ Stir until bubbling, and remove from heat.
- ➢ Stir in the water and vinegar
- ➢ Then bring back to the fire and bring to a boil, stirring constantly
- ➢ Boil and stir.
- ➢ Slowly add bacon and potato slices to the vinegar/water mixture
- ➢ Stir gently until the potatoes are warmed up.

NUTRITION INFORMATION: Calories:205 Fat:6.5g Carbohydrates:32.9g Protein:4.3g Sodium:814mg

156. CHICKEN FIESTA SALAD

Servings: 4   **Cook Time: 20 Min**   **Prep Time 20 Min**

INGREDIENTS:

- ✓ 2 halves of chicken fillet without skin or bones
- ✓ 1 packet of herbs for fajitas, divided
- ✓ 1 tablespoon vegetable oil
- ✓ 1 can black beans, rinsed and drained
- ✓ 1 box of Mexican-style corn

- ✓ 1/2 cup of salsa
- ✓ 1 packet of green salad
- ✓ 1 onion, minced
- ✓ 1 tomato, quartered

DIRECTIONS:

- ➢ Rub the chicken evenly with 1/2 of the herbs for fajitas.
- ➢ Cook the oil in a frying pan over medium heat
- ➢ Cook the chicken for 8 minutes on the side by side or until the juice is clear; put aside.
- ➢ Combine beans, corn, salsa, and other 1/2 fajita spices in a large pan.

- ➢ Heat over medium heat until lukewarm.
- ➢ Prepare the salad by mixing green vegetables, onion, and tomato
- ➢ Cover the chicken salad and dress the beans and corn mixture.

NUTRITION INFORMATION: Calories: 311 Fat:6.4g Carbohydrates:42.2g Protein:23g Sodium:853mg

157. BLACK BEAN & CORN SALAD

Servings: 4   **Cook Time: 0 Min**   **Prep Time 10 Min**

INGREDIENTS:

- ✓ 2 tablespoons vegetable oil
- ✓ 1/4 cup balsamic vinegar
- ✓ 1/2 teaspoon of salt
- ✓ 1/2 teaspoon of white sugar
- ✓ 1/2 teaspoon ground cumin

- ✓ 1/2 teaspoon ground black pepper
- ✓ 1/2 teaspoon chili powder
- ✓ 3 tablespoons chopped fresh coriander
- ✓ 1 can black beans (15 oz)
- ✓ 1 can of sweetened corn (8.75 oz) drained

DIRECTIONS:

- ➤ Combine balsamic vinegar, oil, salt, sugar, black pepper, cumin and chili powder in a small bowl.
- ➤ Combine black corn and beans in a medium bowl.

- ➤ Mix with vinegar and oil vinaigrette
- ➤ Garnish with coriander. Cover and refrigerate overnight.

NUTRITION INFORMATION: Calories: 214 Fat: 8.4g Carbohydrates: 28.6g Protein: 7.5g Sodium: 415mg

158. AWESOME PASTA SALAD

Servings: 16   **Cook Time: 10 Min**   **Prep Time 30 Min**

INGREDIENTS:

- ✓ 1 (16-oz) fusilli pasta package
- ✓ 3 cups of cherry tomatoes
- ✓ 1/2 pound of provolone, diced
- ✓ 1/2 pound of sausage, diced
- ✓ 1/4 pound of pepperoni, cut in half
- ✓ 1 large green pepper
- ✓ 1 can of black olives, drained
- ✓ 1 jar of chilis, drained
- ✓ 1 bottle (8 oz) Italian vinaigrette

DIRECTIONS:

- ➤ Boil a lightly salted water in a pot.
- ➤ Stir in the pasta and cook for about 8 to 10 minutes or until al dente
- ➤ Drain and rinse with cold water.

- ➤ Combine pasta with tomatoes, cheese, salami
- ➤ Add also pepperoni, green pepper, olives, and peppers in a large bowl
- ➤ Pour the vinaigrette and mix well.

NUTRITION INFORMATION: Calories: 310 Fat: 17.7g Carbohydrates: 25.9g Protein: 12.9g Sodium: 746mg

159. SOUTHERN POTATO SALAD

Servings: 4   **Cook Time: 15 Min**   **Prep Time 15 Min**

INGREDIENTS:

- ✓ 4 potatoes
- ✓ 4 eggs
- ✓ 1/2 stalk of celery, finely chopped
- ✓ 1/4 cup sweet taste
- ✓ 1 clove of garlic minced

- ✓ 2 tablespoons mustard
- ✓ 1/2 cup mayonnaise
- ✓ Salt and pepper to taste

DIRECTIONS:

- ➤ Boil water in a pot then situate the potatoes
- ➤ Cook until soft but still firm, about 15 minutes; drain and chop
- ➤ Transfer the eggs in a pan and cover with cold water.
- ➤ Boil the water; cover, remove from heat

- ➤ Let the eggs soak in hot water for 10 minutes
- ➤ Remove then shell and chop.
- ➤ Combine potatoes, eggs, celery, sweet sauce
- ➤ Then garlic, mustard, mayonnaise, salt, and pepper in a large bowl
- ➤ Mix and serve hot.

NUTRITION INFORMATION: Calories: 460 Fat: 27.4g Carbohydrates: 44.6g Protein: 11.3g Sodium: 214mg

160.   SEVEN-LAYER SALAD

Servings: 10   **Cook Time: 5 Min**   **Prep Time 15 Min**

INGREDIENTS:
- ✓ 1-pound bacon
- ✓ 1 head iceberg lettuce 1 red onion, minced
- ✓ 1 pack of 10 frozen peas, thawed
- ✓ 10 oz grated cheddar cheese
- ✓ 1 cup chopped cauliflower
- ✓ 1 1/4 cup mayo
- ✓ 2 tablespoons white sugar
- ✓ 2/3 cup grated Parmesan cheese

DIRECTIONS:
- ➤ Put the bacon in a huge, shallow frying pan
- ➤ Bake over medium heat until smooth. Crumble and set aside.
- ➤ Situate the chopped lettuce in a large bowl and cover with a layer of an onion, peas, grated cheese, cauliflower, and bacon.
- ➤ Prepare the vinaigrette by mixing the mayo, sugar, and parmesan cheese
- ➤ Pour over the salad and cool to cool.

NUTRITION INFORMATION: Calories: 387 Fat: 32.7g Carbohydrates: 9.9g Protein: 14.5g Sodium: 609mg

161.   KALE, QUINOA & AVOCADO SALAD LEMON DIJON VINAIGRETTE

Servings: 4   **Cook Time: 25 Min**   **Prep Time 5 Min**

INGREDIENTS:
- ✓ 2/3 cup of quinoa
- ✓ 1 1/3 cup of water
- ✓ 1 bunch of kale
- ✓ 1/2 avocado, diced and pitted
- ✓ 1/2 cup chopped cucumber
- ✓ 1/3 cup chopped red pepper
- ✓ 2 tablespoons chopped red onion
- ✓ 1 tablespoon of feta crumbled

DIRECTIONS:
- ➤ Boil the quinoa and 1 1/3 cup of water in a pan
- ➤ Adjust heat and simmer until quinoa is tender and water is absorbed for about 15 to 20 minutes
- ➤ Set aside to cool.
- ➤ Place the cabbage in a steam basket over more than an inch of boiling water in a pan
- ➤ Seal the pan with a lid and steam until hot, about 45 seconds
- ➤ Transfer to a large plate
- ➤ Garnish with cabbage, quinoa, avocado, cucumber, pepper, red onion, and feta cheese.
- ➤ Combine olive oil, lemon juice, Dijon mustard, sea salt, and black pepper in a bowl
- ➤ (Until the oil is emulsified in the dressing)
- ➤ Pour over the salad.

NUTRITION INFORMATION: Calories: 342 Fat :20.3g Carbohydrates: 35.4g Protein: 8.9g Sodium: 705mg

162. COBB SALAD

Servings: 6　　　　　　　**Cook Time: 15 Min**　　　　　　**Prep Time 5 Min**

INGREDIENTS:

- ✓ 6 slices of bacon
- ✓ 3 eggs
- ✓ 1 cup Iceberg lettuce, grated
- ✓ 3 cups cooked minced chicken meat
- ✓ 2 tomatoes, seeded and minced

- ✓ 3/4 cup of blue cheese, crumbled
- ✓ 1 avocado - peeled, pitted and diced
- ✓ 3 green onions, minced
- ✓ 1 bottle (8 oz.) Ranch Vinaigrette

DIRECTIONS:

- ➢ Situate the eggs in a pan and soak them completely with cold water
- ➢ Boil the water. Cover and remove from heat
- ➢ Let the eggs rest in hot water for 10 to 12 minutes
- ➢ Remove from hot water, let cool, peel, and chop
- ➢ Situate the bacon in a big, deep frying pan.

- ➢ Bake over medium heat until smooth. Set aside.
- ➢ Divide the grated lettuce into separate plates
- ➢ Spread chicken, eggs, tomatoes, blue cheese, bacon, avocado
- ➢ Then green onions in rows on lettuce
- ➢ Sprinkle with your favorite vinaigrette and enjoy.

NUTRITION INFORMATION: Calories: 525 Fat: 39.9g Carbohydrates: 10.2g Protein: 31.7g sodium: 701mg

163. MEDITERRANEAN VEGGIE BOWL

Servings: 4　　　　　　　**Cook Time: 20 Min**　　　　　　**Prep Time 10 Min**

INGREDIENTS:

- ✓ 1 cup quinoa, rinsed
- ✓ 1½ teaspoons salt, divided
- ✓ 2 cups cherry tomatoes, cut in half

- ✓ 1 large bell pepper, cucumber
- ✓ 1 cup Kalamata olives

DIRECTIONS:

- ➢ Using medium pot over medium heat, boil 2 cups of water
- ➢ Add the bulgur (or quinoa) and 1 teaspoon of salt
- ➢ Cover and cook for 15 to 20 minutes.
- ➢ To arrange the veggies in your 4 bowls, visually divide each bowl into 5 sections
- ➢ Place the cooked bulgur in one section

- ➢ Follow with the tomatoes, bell pepper, cucumbers, and olives
- ➢ Scourge ½ cup of lemon juice, olive oil, remaining ½ teaspoon salt, and black pepper.
- ➢ Evenly spoon the dressing over the 4 bowls.
- ➢ Serve immediately or cover and refrigerate for later.

NUTRITION INFORMATION: Calories: 772 Protein: 6g Carbohydrates: 41g

164. ASIAN SCRAMBLED EGG

Serving: 1　　　　　　　**Cook Time: 10 Min**　　　　　　**Prep Time 10 Min**

INGREDIENTS:

- ✓ 1 large egg
- ✓ 1/2 teaspoons light soy sauce

- ✓ 1/8 teaspoon white pepper
- ✓ 1 tablespoon Olive oil

DIRECTIONS:

- ➢ Beat the eggs in a bowl.
- ➢ To the beaten egg, add soy sauce, one-teaspoon Olive oil, and pepper.
- ➢ Preheat a saucepan on high heat.
- ➢ Add the two tablespoons oil to the saucepan.
- ➢ Then add the mixture of the beaten egg.

- ➢ The edges will begin to cook.
- ➢ Lessen the heat to medium and carefully scramble the eggs.
- ➢ Turn off heat and transfer into a bowl.
- ➢ Serve hot and enjoy

NUTRITION INFORMATION: Calories: 200 Fat: 6.7g Protein: 6.1g Carbohydrates: 1g

165. ARTICHOKE FRITTATAS

Serving: 1   **Cook Time: 30 Min**   **Prep Time 10 Min**

INGREDIENTS:

- ✓ 2.5 oz. dry spinach
- ✓ 1/4 red bell pepper
- ✓ Artichoke (drain the liquid)
- ✓ Green onions
- ✓ Dried tomatoes
- ✓ Two eggs
- ✓ Italian seasoning
- ✓ Salt - Pepper

DIRECTIONS:

- ➢ Preheat oven to medium heat.
- ➢ Brush a bit of oil on the cast-iron skillet.
- ➢ Mix all the vegetables.
- ➢ Add some seasoning.
- ➢ Spread the vegetables evenly in the pan.
- ➢ Whisk the eggs and add some milk.
- ➢ Add some salt and pepper.
- ➢ Mix in some cheese (helps to make it fluffier).
- ➢ Pour the egg mixture in the saucepan.
- ➢ Place the pan inside the oven for about 30 minutes.
- ➢ Enjoy!

NUTRITION INFORMATION: Calories:160 -Protein: 7g -Carbohydrates: 4g -Fat: 3.5g

166. LEAN AND GREEN CHICKEN PESTO PASTA

Serving: 1   **Cook Time: 15 Min**   **Prep Time 5 Min**

INGREDIENTS:

- ✓ 2 cups raw kale leaves
- ✓ 2 tablespoon olive oil
- ✓ 2 cups fresh basil
- ✓ 1/4 teaspoon salt
- ✓ 3 tablespoon lemon juice
- ✓ 3 garlic cloves
- ✓ 2 cups cooked chicken breast
- ✓ 1 cup baby spinach
- ✓ 6 oz. uncooked chicken pasta
- ✓ 3 oz. diced fresh mozzarella
- ✓ Basil leaves or red pepper flakes to garnish

DIRECTIONS:

- ✓ Start by making the pesto, add the kale, lemon juice, basil, garlic cloves, olive oil
- ✓ Then salt to a blender and blend until it is smooth.
- ✓ Add pepper to taste.
- ✓ Cook the pasta and strain off the water
- ✓ Reserve 1/4 cup of the liquid.
- ✓ Get a bowl and mix everything, the cooked pasta, pesto, diced chicken, spinach
- ✓ Add mozzarella, and the reserved pasta liquid.
- ✓ Sprinkle the mixture with additional chopped basil or red paper flakes (optional).
- ✓ Now your salad is ready.
- ✓ Serve it warm or chilled.
- ✓ (Also, it can be taken as a salad mix-ins or as a side dish. Leftovers should be stored in the refrigerator inside an air-tight container for 3–5 days)

NUTRITION INFORMATION: Calories:244 -Protein: 20.5g -Carbohydrates: 22.5g -Fats: 10g

167. MOSTO CARAMELIZED ONIONS

Servings: 10   **Cook Time: 20 Min**   **Prep Time 5 Min**

INGREDIENTS:
- ✓ Onion slices - 1 cup
- ✓ Chicken broth (low sodium) - 1/4 cup
- ✓ Balsamic mosto cotto (or use a balsamic reduction - do not use vinegar) - 4 tablespoon
- ✓ Pinch of sea salt and fresh peppercorns

DIRECTIONS:
- ➢ Add the broth and onions to your pan
- ➢ Cook on a stove over a medium heat for about 20 minutes.
- ➢ Without getting brown, once the onions become soft with the liquid evaporated
- ➢ Add the balsamic to the pan.
- ➢ Turn of the stove and allow the pan on the stove
- ➢ Stir gently and allow the onions to steep into the balsamic.
- ➢ Then serve.
- ➢ It can be stored in a refrigerator for up to 1 week.

NUTRITION INFORMATION: Calories:6 -Fats: 0g -Carbs: 1.4g -Fiber: 0.2g -Sugar: 0.8g -Protein: 0.1g

168. PORK LOIN CARAMELIZED ONIONS

Servings: 4   **Cook Time: 25 Min**   **Prep Time 5 Min**

INGREDIENTS:
- ➢ Seasoning mix (or use a mixture of any of garlic, black pepper, salt, onion and parsley) - 1 teaspoons
- ➢ Pork tenderloin (you can use chicken breasts or beef tenderloin)- 1 1/2 lbs.

DIRECTIONS:
- ➢ Preheat your oven to 400.
- ➢ Season both sides of the tenderloin.
- ➢ Over high heat, place the oven-safe pan on your oven
- ➢ Grease it with nonstick cooking spray.
- ➢ Once heated up, place the tenderloins in the pan without touching each other.
- ➢ Cook each side for about 3 minutes, or until it turns brown.
- ➢ Transfer the tenderloins to the oven
- ➢ Allow to cook for about
- ➢ 25 minutes or until well cooked.
- ➢ Remove from heat and allow it to cool down a bit for about 3 minutes.
- ➢ Slice the pork.
- ➢ Meanwhile, prepare the balsamic caramelize onions
- ➢ Serve with the sliced pork.

NUTRITION INFORMATION: Calories:220 -Fats: 5g -Carbs: 3.8g -Fiber: 0.9g -Sugar: 1.7g -Protein: 37.5g

169. SUNRISE SALMON

Servings: 4 **Cook Time: 15 Min** **Prep Time 15 Min**

INGREDIENTS:

- ✓ Wild caught salmon filet (will cook best if you have it at room temp) - 1 1/2 pounds
- ✓ Sunrise seasoning (or use a mixture of cumin, paprika, salt, cayenne, pepper, garlic, and onion to taste) - 1 tablespoon

DIRECTIONS:

- ➤ Preheat your nonstick pan for about 1minutesute over high heat.
- ➤ Meanwhile, sprinkle the seasoning   on the salmon. Don't sprinkle on the skin side.
- ➤ Low the heat to medium-high heat.
- ➤ With the seasoned side down, place the salmon on the pan
- ➤ Cook for about 6 minutes.
- ➤ Lower the heat further to medium-low and flip the salmon.
- ➤ Cook for extra 6 minutes.
- ➤ Serve

NUTRITION INFORMATION: Calories:192 -Fats: 8.8g -Carbs: 0.8g -Fiber: 0g -Sugar: 0.2g -Protein: 27.5g

170. GREEN BEANS GARLIC

Servings: 4 **Cook Time: 10 Min** **Prep Time 5 Min**

INGREDIENTS:

- ✓ Green beans (with ends trimmed) - 1 1/2 pounds
- ✓ Garlic and spring onion seasoning (or use a mixture of pepper, fresh chopped garlic, and salt) - 1/2 tablespoon
- ✓ Roasted garlic oil (or any other oil you like) - 1tablespoon
- ✓ Parmesan cheese (freshly grated) - 4 tablespoons

DIRECTIONS:

- ➤ Add the green beans to a pot.
- ➤ Add up to 1 inch of water to the pot.
- ➤ Sprinkle over with the seasoning.
- ➤ Cover the pot and place it on your stove.
- ➤ Cook over high heat and bring to boil, about 7 minutes
- ➤ (Or until the beans steams and becomes crisp tender)
- ➤ Drain the water and drizzle over with the garlic oil and pepper and salt.
- ➤ Sprinkle over with the Parmesan cheese.
- ➤ Serve.

NUTRITION INFORMATION: Calories: 84 -Fats: 5g -Carbs: 7.8g -Fiber: 3.7g -Sugar: 1.5g -Protein: 4g

171. GRILLED LEMON SHRIMP

Servings: 6 **Cook Time: 5 Min** **Prep Time 20 Min**

INGREDIENTS:

- ✓ 2 tablespoons garlic, minced
- ✓ ½ cup lemon juice
- ✓ 3 tablespoons fresh Italian parsley, finely chopped
- ✓ ¼ cup extra-virgin olive oil
- ✓ 1 teaspoon salt
- ✓ 2 pounds (907 g) jumbo shrimp (21 to 25), peeled and deveined

DIRECTIONS:

- ➤ In a large bowl, mix the garlic, lemon juice, parsley, olive oil, and salt.
- ➤ Add the shrimp to the bowl
- ➤ Toss to make sure all the pieces are coated with the marinade
- ➤ Let the shrimp sit for 15 minutes.
- ➤ Preheat a grill, grill pan, or lightly oiled skillet to high heat
- ➤ While heating, thread about 5 to 6 pieces of shrimp onto each skewer.
- ➤ Place the skewers on the grill, grill pan, or skillet
- ➤ Cook for 2 to 3 minutes on each side
- ➤ (Until cooked through)
- ➤ Serve warm.

NUTRITION INFORMATION: Calories:402 fat: 18g protein: 57g carbs: 4g fiber: 0g sodium: 1224mg

172. ITALIAN FRIED SHRIMP

Servings: 4   **Cook Time: 5 Min**   **Prep Time 10 Min**

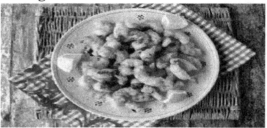

INGREDIENTS:

- ✓ 2 large eggs
- ✓ 2 cups seasoned Italian bread crumbs 1 teaspoon salt
- ✓ 1 cup flour
- ✓ 1 pound (454 g) large shrimp (21 to 25), peeled and deveined
- ✓ Extra-virgin olive oil

DIRECTIONS:

- ➤ In a small bowl, beat the eggs with 1 tablespoon water
- ➤ Then transfer to a shallow dish.
- ➤ Add the bread crumbs and salt to a separate shallow dish; mix well.
- ➤ Place the flour into a third shallow dish.
- ➤ Coat the shrimp in the flour, then egg, and finally the bread crumbs

- ➤ Place on a plate and repeat with all of the shrimp.
- ➤ Preheat a skillet over high heat
- ➤ Pour in enough olive oil to coat the bottom of the skillet
- ➤ Cook the shrimp in the hot skillet for 2 to 3 minutes on each side
- ➤ Take the shrimp out and drain on a paper towel. Serve warm.

NUTRITION INFORMATION: Calories: 714 fat: 34g protein: 37g carbs: 63g fiber: 3g sodium: 1727mg

173. COD SAFFRON RICE

Servings: 4   **Cook Time: 35 Min**   **Prep Time 10 Min**

INGREDIENTS:

- ✓ 4 tablespoons extra-virgin olive oil, divided
- ✓ 1 large onion, chopped
- ✓ 3 cod fillets, rinsed and patted dry
- ✓ 4½ cups water

- ✓ 1 teaspoon saffron threads
- ✓ 1½ teaspoons salt
- ✓ 1 teaspoon turmeric
- ✓ Cups long-grain rice, rinsed

DIRECTIONS:

- ➤ In a large pot over medium heat, cook 2 tablespoons of olive oil and the onions for 5 minutes.
- ➤ While the onions are cooking, preheat another large pan over high heat
- ➤ Add the remaining 2 tablespoons of olive oil and the cod fillets
- ➤ Cook the cod for 2 minutes on each side,
- ➤ Then remove from the pan and set aside.
- ➤ Once the onions are done cooking

- ➤ Then the water, saffron, salt, turmeric, and rice, stirring to combine
- ➤ Cover and cook for 12 minutes.
- ➤ Cut the cod up into 1-inch pieces
- ➤ Place the cod pieces in the rice
- ➤ Lightly toss, cover, and cook for another 10 minutes.
- ➤ Once the rice is done cooking, fluff with a fork
- ➤ Cover, and let stand for 5 minutes. Serve warm.

NUTRITION INFORMATION: Calories: 564 fat: 15g protein: 26g carbs: 78g fiber: 2g sodium: 945mg

174.   THYME WHOLE ROASTED RED SNAPPER

Servings: 4   **Cook Time: 45 Min**   **Prep Time 5 Min**

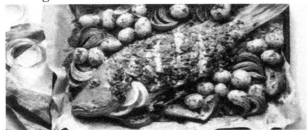

INGREDIENTS:

- ✓ 1 (2 to 2½ pounds / 907 g to 1.1 kg) whole red snapper, cleaned and scaled
- ✓ 2 lemons, sliced (about 10 slices)
- ✓ 3 cloves garlic, sliced
- ✓ 4 or 5 sprigs of thyme
- ✓ 3 tablespoons cold salted butter, cut into small cubes, divided (optional)

DIRECTIONS:

- ➢ Preheat the oven to 350°F (180°C).
- ➢ Cut a piece of foil to about the size of your baking sheet
- ➢ Put the foil on the baking sheet.
- ➢ Make a horizontal slice through the belly of the fish to create a pocket.
- ➢ Place 3 slices of lemon on the foil and the fish on top of the lemons.
- ➢ Stuff the fish with the garlic, thyme, 3 lemon slices and butter
- ➢ Reserve 3 pieces of butter.
- ➢ Place the reserved 3 pieces of butter on top of the fish, and 3 or 4 slices of lemon on top of the butter
- ➢ Bring the foil together and seal it to make a pocket around the fish.
- ➢ Put the fish in the oven
- ➢ Bake for 45 minutes
- ➢ Serve with remaining fresh lemon slices.

NUTRITION INFORMATION: Calories: 345 fat: 13g protein: 54g carbs: 12g fiber: 3g sodium: 170mg

175.   CILANTRO LEMON SHRIMP

Servings: 4   **Cook Time: 10 Min**   **Prep Time 20 Min**

INGREDIENTS:

- ✓ ⅓ cup lemon juice
- ✓ 4 garlic cloves
- ✓ 1 cup fresh cilantro leaves
- ✓ ½ teaspoon ground coriander
- ✓ 3 tablespoons extra-virgin olive oil
- ✓ 1 teaspoon salt
- ✓ 1½ pounds (680 g) large shrimp (21 to 25), deveined and shells removed

DIRECTIONS:

- ➢ In a food processor, pulse the lemon juice
- ➢ Then garlic, cilantro, coriander, olive oil, and salt 10 times.
- ➢ Put the shrimp in a bowl or plastic zip-top bag
- ➢ Pour in the cilantro marinade, and let sit for 15 minutes.
- ➢ Preheat a skillet on high heat.
- ➢ Put the shrimp and marinade in the skillet
- ➢ Cook the shrimp for 3 minutes on each side. Serve warm.

NUTRITION INFORMATION: Calories: 225 fat: 12g protein: 28g carbs: 5g fiber: 1g sodium: 763mg

176. SEAFOOD RISOTTO

Servings: 4   **Cook Time: 30 Min**   **Prep Time 10 Min**

INGREDIENTS:
- ✓ 6 cups vegetable broth
- ✓ 3 tablespoons extra-virgin olive oil
- ✓ 1 large onion, chopped
- ✓ 3 cloves garlic, minced
- ✓ ½ teaspoon saffron threads
- ✓ 1½ cups arborio rice
- ✓ 1½ teaspoons salt
- ✓ 8 ounces (227 g) shrimp (21 to 25), peeled and deveined
- ✓ 8 ounces (227 g) scallops

DIRECTIONS:
- ➤ In a large saucepan over medium heat, bring the broth to a low simmer.
- ➤ In a large skillet over medium heat
- ➤ Cook the olive oil, onion, garlic, and saffron for 3 minutes.
- ➤ Add the rice, salt, and 1 cup of the broth to the skillet
- ➤ Stir the ingredients together
- ➤ Cook over low heat until most of the liquid is absorbed
- ➤ Repeat steps with broth, adding ½ cup of broth at a time
- ➤ Cook until all but ½ cup of the broth is absorbed.
- ➤ Add the shrimp and scallops when you stir in the final ½ cup of broth
- ➤ Cover and let cook for 10 minutes. Serve warm.

NUTRITION INFORMATION: Calories: 460 fat: 12g protein: 24g carbs: 64g fiber: 2g sodium: 2432mg

177. GARLIC SHRIMP BLACK BEAN PASTA

Servings: 4   **Cook Time: 15 Min**   **Prep Time 10 Min**

INGREDIENTS:
- ✓ 1 pound (454 g) black bean linguine or spaghetti
- ✓ 1 pound (454 g) fresh shrimp, peeled and deveined
- ✓ 4 tablespoons extra-virgin olive oil
- ✓ 1 onion, finely chopped
- ✓ 3 garlic cloves, minced
- ✓ ¼ cup basil, cut into strips

DIRECTIONS:
- ➤ Bring a large pot of water to a boil and cook the pasta according to the package instructions.
- ➤ In the last 5 minutes of cooking the pasta, add the shrimp to the hot water
- ➤ Allow them to cook for 3 to 5 minutes
- ➤ Once they turn pink, take them out of the hot water,
- ➤ (If they are overcooked, pass them under cold water).
- ➤ Set aside.
- ➤ Reserve 1 cup of the pasta cooking water and drain the noodles
- ➤ In the same pan, heat the oil over medium-high heat and cook the onion and garlic for 7 to 10 minutes. Once the onion is translucent, add the pasta back in and toss well.
- ➤ Plate the pasta, then top with shrimp and garnish with basil.

NUTRITION INFORMATION: Calories: 668 fat: 19g protein: 57g carbs: 73g fiber: 31g sodium: 615mg

178. FAST SEAFOOD PAELLA

Servings: 4   **Cook Time: 20 Min**   **Prep Time 20 Min**

INGREDIENTS:

- ¼ cup plus 1 tablespoon extra-virgin olive oil
- 1 large onion, finely chopped
- 2 tomatoes, peeled and chopped
- 1½ tablespoons garlic powder
- 1½ cups medium-grain Spanish paella rice or arborio rice
- 2 carrots, finely diced
- Salt, to taste
- 1 tablespoon sweet paprika
- 8 ounces (227 g) lobster meat or canned crab
- ½ cup frozen peas
- 3 cups chicken stock, plus more if needed
- 1 cup dry white wine
- 6 jumbo shrimp, unpeeled
- ⅓ pound (136 g) calamari rings
- 1 lemon, halved

DIRECTIONS:

- In a large sauté pan or skillet (16-inch is ideal), heat the oil over medium heat
- (Until small bubbles start to escape from oil)
- Add the onion and cook for about 3 minutes, until fragrant
- Then add tomatoes and garlic powder
- Cook for 5 to 10 minutes
- (Until the tomatoes are reduced by half and the consistency is sticky)
- Stir in the rice, carrots, salt, paprika, lobster, and peas and mix well
- In a pot or microwave-safe bowl, heat the chicken stock to almost boiling
- Then add it to the rice mixture. Bring to a simmer, then add the wine.
- Smooth out the rice in the bottom of the pan
- Cover and cook on low for 10 minutes, mixing occasionally, to prevent burning.
- Top the rice with the shrimp, cover
- Cook for 5 more minutes
- Add additional broth to the pan if the rice looks dried out.
- Right before removing the skillet from the heat, add the calamari rings
- Toss the ingredients frequently
- In about 2 minutes, the rings will look opaque
- Remove the pan from the heat immediately
- (If you don't want the paella to overcook)
- Squeeze fresh lemon juice over the dish.

NUTRITION INFORMATION: Calories: 632 fat: 20g protein: 34g carbs: 71g fiber: 5g sodium: 920mg

179. CRISPY FRIED SARDINES

Servings: 4   **Cook Time: 5 Min**   **Prep Time 5 Min**

INGREDIENTS:

- Avocado oil, as needed
- 1½ pounds (680 g) whole fresh sardines, scales removed
- 1 teaspoon salt
- 1 teaspoon freshly ground black pepper
- 2 cups flour

DIRECTIONS:

- Preheat a deep skillet over medium heat
- Pour in enough oil so there is about 1 inch of it in the pan.
- Season the fish with the salt and pepper.
- Dredge the fish in the flour so it is completely covered.
- Slowly drop in 1 fish at a time, making sure not to overcrowd the pan.
- Cook for about 3 minutes on each side
- (Or just until the fish begins to brown on all sides)
- Serve warm.

NUTRITION INFORMATION: Calories: 794 fat: 47g protein: 48g carbs: 44g fiber: 2g sodium: 1441mg

180. ORANGE ROASTED SALMON

Servings: 4   **Cook Time: 25 Min**   **Prep Time 10 Min**

INGREDIENTS:

- ½ cup extra-virgin olive oil, divided
- 2 tablespoons balsamic vinegar
- 2 tablespoons garlic powder, divided
- 1 tablespoon cumin seeds
- 1 teaspoon sea salt, divided
- 1 teaspoon freshly ground black pepper, divided
- 2 teaspoons smoked paprika
- 4 (8-ounce / 227-g) salmon fillets, skinless
- 2 small red onion, thinly sliced
- ½ cup halved Campari tomatoes

- 1 small fennel bulb, thinly sliced lengthwise
- 1 large carrot, thinly sliced
- 8 medium portobello mushrooms
- 8 medium radishes, sliced ⅛ inch thick
- ½ cup dry white wine
- ½ lime, zested
- Handful cilantro leaves
- ½ cup halved pitted Kalamata olives
- 1 orange, thinly sliced
- 4 roasted sweet potatoes, cut in wedges lengthwise

DIRECTIONS:

- Preheat the oven to 375°F (190°C).
- In a medium bowl, mix 6 tablespoons of olive oil, the balsamic vinegar, 1 tablespoon of garlic powder
- Then the cumin seeds, ¼ teaspoon of sea salt, ¼ teaspoon of pepper, and the paprika
- Put the salmon in the bowl and marinate while preparing the vegetables, about 10 minutes.
- Heat an oven-safe sauté pan or skillet on medium-high heat
- Sear the top of the salmon for about 2 minutes (Or until lightly brown) Set aside.
- Add the remaining 2 tablespoons of olive oil to the same skillet
- Once it's hot, add the onion, tomatoes, fennel, carrot, mushrooms, radishes

- Join also the remaining 1 teaspoon of garlic powder, ¾ teaspoon of salt, and ¾ teaspoon of pepper
- Mix well and cook for 5 to 7 minutes, until fragrant. Add wine and mix well.
- Place the salmon on top of the vegetable mixture, browned-side up
- Sprinkle the fish with lime zest and cilantro and place the olives around the fish
- Put orange slices over the fish and cook for about 7 additional minutes
- While this is baking, add the sliced sweet potato wedges on a baking sheet
- Bake this alongside the skillet.
- Remove from the oven, cover the skillet tightly
- Let rest for about 3 minutes.

NUTRITION INFORMATION: Calories: 841 fat: 41g protein: 59g carbs: 60g fiber: 15g sodium: 908mg

181. LEMON ROSEMARY BRANZINO

Servings: 2   **Cook Time: 30 Min**   **Prep Time 15 Min**

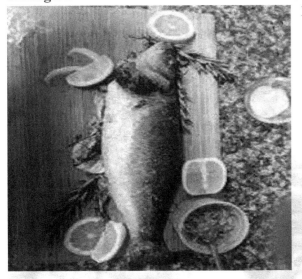

INGREDIENTS:

- ✓ 4 tablespoons extra-virgin olive oil, divided
- ✓ 2 (8-ounce / 227-g) branzino fillets, preferably at least 1 inch thick
- ✓ 1 garlic clove, minced
- ✓ 1 bunch scallions, white part only, thinly sliced
- ✓ ½ cup sliced pitted Kalamata or other good-quality black olives
- ✓ 1 large carrot, cut into ¼-inch rounds
- ✓ 10 to 12 small cherry tomatoes, halved
- ✓ ½ cup dry white wine
- ✓ 2 tablespoons paprika
- ✓ 2 teaspoons kosher salt
- ✓ ½ tablespoon ground chili pepper, preferably Turkish or Aleppo
- ✓ 2 rosemary sprigs or 1 tablespoon dried rosemary
- ✓ small lemon, very thinly sliced

DIRECTIONS:

- ➤ Warm a large, oven-safe sauté pan or skillet over high heat until hot, about 2 minutes
- ➤ Carefully add 1 tablespoon of olive oil and heat until it shimmers, 10 to 15 seconds
- ➤ Brown the branzino fillets for 2 minutes, skin-side up
- ➤ Carefully flip the fillets skin-side down
- ➤ Cook for another 2 minutes, until browned. Set aside.
- ➤ Swirl 2 tablespoons of olive oil around the skillet to coat evenly
- ➤ Add the garlic, scallions, kalamata olives, carrot, and tomatoes

- ➤ Let the vegetables sauté for 5 minutes, until softened
- ➤ Add the wine, stirring until all ingredients are well integrated
- ➤ Carefully place the fish over the sauce.
- ➤ Preheat the oven to 450°F (235°C).
- ➤ While the oven is heating, brush the fillets with 1 tablespoon of olive oil
- ➤ Season with paprika, salt, and chili pepper
- ➤ Top each fillet with a rosemary sprig and several slices of lemon
- ➤ Scatter the olives over fish and around the pan.
- ➤ Roast until lemon slices are browned or singed, about 10 minutes

NUTRITION INFORMATION: Calories: 725 fat: 43g protein: 58g carbs: 25g fiber: 10g sodium: 2954mg

182. GRILLED VEGGIE AND HUMMUS WRAP

Servings: 6   **Cook Time: 10 Min**   **Prep Time 15 Min**

INGREDIENTS:

- ✓ 1 large eggplant
- ✓ 1 large onion
- ✓ ½ cup extra-virgin olive oil
- ✓ 6 lavash wraps or large pita bread
- ✓ 1 cup Creamy Traditional Hummus

DIRECTIONS:

- ➢ Preheat a grill, large grill pan, or lightly oiled large skillet on medium heat.
- ➢ Slice the eggplant and onion into circles
- ➢ Rub the vegetables with olive oil and sprinkle with salt.
- ➢ Cook the vegetables on both sides, about 3 to 4 minutes each side.
- ➢ To make the wrap, lay the lavash or pita flat
- ➢ Spread about 2 tablespoons of hummus on the wrap.
- ➢ Evenly divide the vegetables among the wraps
- ➢ Lay them along one side of the wrap
- ➢ Gently fold over the side of the wrap with the vegetables
- ➢ Tucking them in and making a tight wrap.
- ➢ Lay the wrap seam side-down and cut in half or thirds.
- ➢ You can also wrap each sandwich with plastic wrap to help it hold its shape and eat it later.

NUTRITION INFORMATION: Calories: 362 Protein: 15g Carbohydrates: 28g

183. ANCHOVY AND ORANGE SALAD

Servings: 4   **Cook Time: 0 Min**   **Prep Time 10 Min**

INGREDIENTS:

- ✓ 1 small red onion, sliced into thin rounds
- ✓ 1 tbsp fresh lemon juice
- ✓ 1/8 tsp pepper or more to taste
- ✓ 16 oil cure Kalamata olives
- ✓ 2 tsp finely minced fennel fronds for garnish
- ✓ 3 tbsp extra virgin olive oil
- ✓ 4 small oranges, preferably blood oranges
- ✓ 6 anchovy fillets

DIRECTIONS:

- ✓ With a paring knife, peel oranges including the membrane that surrounds it
- ✓ In a plate, slice oranges into thin circles
- ✓ Allow plate to catch the orange juices
- ✓ On serving plate, arrange orange slices on a layer
- ✓ Sprinkle oranges with onion, followed by olives and then anchovy fillets
- ✓ Drizzle with oil, lemon juice and orange juice
- ✓ Sprinkle with pepper
- ✓ Allow salad to stand for 30 minutes at room temperature to allow the flavors to develop
- ✓ To serve, garnish with fennel fronds and enjoy.

NUTRITION INFORMATION: Calories: 133.9; Protein: 3.2 g; Carbs: 14.3g; Fat: 7.1g

184. SPANAKOPITA DIP

Servings: 2   **Cook Time: 14 Min**   **Prep Time 15 Min**

INGREDIENTS:

- ✓ Olive oil cooking spray
- ✓ 3 tablespoons olive oil, divided
- ✓ 2 tablespoons minced white onion
- ✓ 2 garlic cloves, minced
- ✓ 4 cups fresh spinach
- ✓ 4 ounces (113 g) cream cheese, softened
- ✓ 4 ounces (113 g) feta cheese, divided Zest of

- ✓ 1 lemon
- ✓ ¼ teaspoon ground nutmeg
- ✓ 1 teaspoon dried dill
- ✓ ½ teaspoon salt
- ✓ Pita chips, carrot sticks, or sliced bread for serving (optional)

DIRECTIONS:

- ➤ Preheat the air fryer to 360°F (182°C)
- ➤ Coat the inside of a 6-inch ramekin or baking dish with olive oil cooking spray.
- ➤ In a large skillet over medium heat, heat 1 tablespoon of the olive oil
- ➤ Add the onion, then cook for 1 minute.
- ➤ Then in the garlic and cook, stirring for 1 minute more.
- ➤ Reduce the heat to low and mix in the spinach and water
- ➤ Let this cook for 2 to 3 minutes, or until the spinach has wilted
- ➤ Remove the skillet from the heat.

- ➤ In a medium bowl, combine the cream cheese, 2 ounces of the feta
- ➤ Add the remaining 2 tablespoons of olive oil, along with the lemon zest, nutmeg, dill, and salt
- ➤ Mix until just combined.
- ➤ Join alsoAdd the vegetables to the cheese base and stir until combined
- ➤ Pour the dip mixture into the prepared ramekin
- ➤ Top with the remaining 2 ounces of feta cheese.
- ➤ Place the dip into the air fryer basket and cook for 10 minutes
- ➤ (Or until heated through and bubbling)
- ➤ Serve with pita chips, carrot sticks, or sliced bread

NUTRITION INFORMATION: Calories: 550 fat: 52g protein: 14g carbs: 9g fiber: 2g sodium: 113mg

185. ASIAN PEANUT SAUCE OVER NOODLE SALAD

Servings: 4   **Cook Time: 0 Min**   **Prep Time 10 Min**

INGREDIENTS:

- ✓ 1 cup shredded green cabbage
- ✓ 1 cup shredded red cabbage
- ✓ 1/4 cup chopped
- ✓ Cilantro

- ✓ 1/4 cup chopped peanuts
- ✓ 1/4 cup chopped scallions
- ✓ 4 cups shiritake noodles (drained and rinsed)

ASIAN PEANUT SAUCE INGREDIENTS:

- ✓ ¼ cup sugar free peanut butter
- ✓ ¼ teaspoon cayenne pepper
- ✓ ½ cup filtered water
- ✓ ½ teaspoon kosher salt
- ✓ 1 tablespoon fish sauce (or coconut aminos for vegan)

- ✓ 1 tablespoon granulated erythritol sweetener
- ✓ 1 tablespoon lime juice
- ✓ 1 tablespoon toasted sesame oil
- ✓ 1 tablespoon wheat-free soy sauce
- ✓ 1 teaspoon minced garlic
- ✓ 2 tablespoons minced ginger

DIRECTIONS:

- ➤ In a large salad bowl, combine all noodle salad ingredients
- ➤ Toss well to mix. In a blender

- ➤ Mix all sauce ingredients and pulse until smooth and creamy
- ➤ Pour sauce over the salad and toss well to coat
- ➤ Evenly divide into four equal servings and enjoy.

NUTRITION INFORMATION: Calories: 104; Protein: 7.0g; Carbs: 12.0g; Fat: 16.0g

186. SPANISH GREEN BEANS

Servings: 4　　　　**Cook Time: 20 Min**　　　　**Prep Time 10 Min**

INGREDIENTS:
- ✓ 1 large onion, chopped
- ✓ 4 cloves garlic, finely chopped
- ✓ 1-pound green beans, fresh or frozen, trimmed
- ✓ 1 (15-ounce) can diced tomatoes

DIRECTIONS:
- ➢ In a huge pot over medium heat, cook olive oil, onion, and garlic; cook for 1 minute.
- ➢ Cut the green beans into 2-inch pieces.
- ➢ Add the green beans and 1 teaspoon of salt to the pot and toss everything together
- ➢ Cook for 3 minutes.
- ➢ Add the diced tomatoes, remaining ½ teaspoon of salt, and black pepper to the pot
- ➢ Continue to cook for another 12 minutes, stirring occasionally.
- ➢ Serve warm

NUTRITION INFORMATION: Calories: 200 Protein: 4g Carbohydrates: 18g

187. RUSTIC CAULIFLOWER AND CARROT HASH

Servings: 4　　　　**Cook Time: 10 Min**　　　　**Prep Time 10 Min**

INGREDIENTS:
- ✓ 1 large onion, chopped
- ✓ 1 tablespoon garlic, minced
- ✓ 2 cups carrots, diced
- ✓ 4 cups cauliflower pieces, washed
- ✓ ½ teaspoon ground cumin

DIRECTIONS:
- ➢ In a big frying pan on medium heat
- ➢ Heat up 3 tbsps. of olive oil, onion, garlic, and carrots for 3 minutes.
- ➢ Cut the cauliflower into 1-inch or bite-size pieces
- ➢ Add the cauliflower, salt, and cumin to the skillet
- ➢ Toss to combine with the carrots and onions.
- ➢ Cover and cook for 3 minutes.
- ➢ Throw the vegetables and continue to cook uncovered for an additional 3 to 4 minutes.
- ➢ Serve warm.

NUTRITION INFORMATION: Calories: 159 Protein: 3g Carbohydrates: 15g

188. ROASTED CAULIFLOWER AND TOMATOES

Servings: 4   **Cook Time: 25 Min**   **Prep Time 5 Min**

INGREDIENTS:

- ✓ 4 cups cauliflower, cut into
- ✓ 1-inch pieces
- ✓ 6 tablespoons extra-virgin olive oil, divided
- ✓ 4 cups cherry tomatoes
- ✓ ½ teaspoon freshly ground black pepper
- ✓ ½ cup grated Parmesan cheese

DIRECTIONS:

- ➢ Preheat the oven to 425°F.
- ➢ Add the cauliflower, 3 tablespoons of olive oil, and ½ teaspoon of salt to a large bowl
- ➢ Toss to evenly coat. Pour onto a baking sheet and spread the cauliflower out in an even layer.
- ➢ In another large bowl, add the tomatoes, remaining 3 tablespoons of olive oil, and ½ teaspoon of salt, and toss to coat evenly
- ➢ Pour onto a different baking sheet.
- ➢ Put the sheet of cauliflower and the sheet of tomatoes in the oven to roast for 17 to 20 minutes
- ➢ (Until the cauliflower is lightly browned and tomatoes are plump)
- ➢ Using a spatula, spoon the cauliflower into a serving dish
- ➢ Top with tomatoes, black pepper, and Parmesan cheese
- ➢ Serve warm.

NUTRITION INFORMATION: Calories: 294 Protein: 9g Carbohydrates: 13g

189. ROASTED ACORN SQUASH

Servings: 6   **Cook Time: 35 Min**   **Prep Time 10 Min**

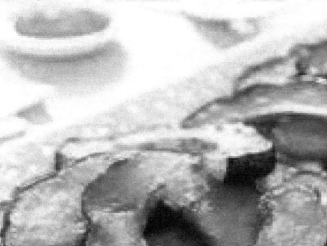

INGREDIENTS:

- ✓ 2 acorn squash, medium to large
- ✓ 2 tablespoons extra-virgin olive oil
- ✓ 5 tablespoons unsalted butter
- ✓ ¼ cup chopped sage leaves
- ✓ 2 tablespoons fresh thyme leaves

DIRECTIONS:

- ➢ Preheat the oven to 400°F.
- ➢ Cut the acorn squash in half lengthwise. Scoop out the seeds and cut it horizontally into ¾-inch-thick slices.
- ➢ In a large bowl, drizzle the squash with the olive oil
- ➢ Sprinkle with salt, and toss together to coat.
- ➢ Lay the acorn squash flat on a baking sheet.
- ➢ Put the baking sheet in the oven and bake the squash for 20 minutes
- ➢ Flip squash over with a spatula and bake for another 15 minutes.
- ➢ Melt the butter in a medium saucepan over medium heat.
- ➢ Add the sage and thyme to the melted butter and let them cook for 30 seconds.
- ➢ Transfer the cooked squash slices to a plate
- ➢ Spoon the butter/herb mixture over the squash
- ➢ Season with salt and black pepper. Serve warm.

NUTRITION INFORMATION: Calories: 188 Protein: 1g Carbohydrates: 16g

190. SAUTÉED GARLIC SPINACH

Servings: 4   **Cook Time: 10 Min**   **Prep Time 15 Min**

INGREDIENTS:

- ✓ ¼ cup extra-virgin olive oil
- ✓ 1 large onion, thinly sliced
- ✓ 3 cloves garlic, minced
- ✓ 6 (1-pound) bags of baby spinach, washed
- ✓ 1 lemon, cut into wedges

DIRECTIONS:

- ➢ Cook the olive oil, onion, and garlic in a large skillet for 2 minutes over medium heat.
- ➢ Add one bag of spinach and ½ teaspoon of salt
- ➢ Cover the skillet and let the spinach wilt for 30 seconds
- ➢ Repeat (omitting the salt), adding 1 bag of spinach at a time.
- ➢ Once all the spinach has been added
- ➢ Remove the cover and cook for 3 minutes, letting some of the moisture evaporate.
- ➢ Serve warm with lemon juice over the top

NUTRITION INFORMATION: Calories: 301 Protein: 17g Carbohydrates: 29g

191. CHICKEN BREAST SOUP

Servings: 4   **Cook Time: 4 H**   **Prep Time 5 Min**

INGREDIENTS:

- ✓ 3 chicken breasts, skinless, boneless, cubed
- ✓ 2 celery stalks, chopped
- ✓ 2 carrots, chopped
- ✓ 2 tablespoons olive oil 1 red onion, chopped
- ✓ 3 garlic cloves, minced 4 cups chicken stock
- ✓ 1 tablespoon parsley, chopped

DIRECTIONS:

- ➢ In your slow cooker, mix all the ingredients except the parsley
- ➢ Cover and cook on High for 4 hours.
- ➢ Add the parsley, stir, ladle the soup into bowls and serve

NUTRITION INFORMATION: Calories: 445 Fat: 21.1g Fiber: 1.6g Carbs: 7.4g Protein:54.3g

192. CAULIFLOWER CURRY

Servings: 4   **Cook Time: 5 H**   **Prep Time 5 Min**

INGREDIENTS:

- ✓ 1 cauliflower head, florets separated
- ✓ 2 carrots, sliced
- ✓ 1 red onion, chopped
- ✓ ¾ cup coconut milk
- ✓ 2 garlic cloves, minced
- ✓ 2 tablespoons curry powder
- ✓ A pinch of salt and black pepper
- ✓ 1 tablespoon red pepper flakes
- ✓ 1 teaspoon garam masala

DIRECTIONS:

- ➢ In your slow cooker, mix all the ingredients.
- ➢ Cover, cook on high for 5 hours, divide into bowls and serve.

NUTRITION INFORMATION: Calories: 160 Fat: 11.5g Fiber: 5.4g Carbs: 14.7g Protein: 3.6g

193. BALELA SALAD FROM THE MIDDLE EAST

Servings: 6   **Cook Time: 0 Min**   **Prep Time 10 Min**

INGREDIENTS:

- ✓ 1 jalapeno, finely chopped (optional)
- ✓ 1/2 green bell pepper, cored and chopped
- ✓ 2 1/2 cups grape tomatoes, slice in halves
- ✓ 1/2 cup sun-dried tomatoes
- ✓ 1/2 cup freshly chopped parsley leaves
- ✓ 1/2 cup freshly chopped mint or basil leaves

- ✓ 1/3 cup pitted Kalamata olives
- ✓ 1/4 cup pitted green olives
- ✓ 3 1/2 cups cooked chickpeas, drained and rinsed
- ✓ 3–5 green onions, both white and green parts, chopped

DRESSING INGREDIENTS:

- ✓ 1 garlic clove, minced
- ✓ 1 tsp ground sumac
- ✓ 1/2 tsp Aleppo pepper
- ✓ 1/4 cup Early Harvest Greek extra virgin olive oil
- ✓ 1/4 to 1/2 tsp crushed red pepper (optional)

- ✓ 2 tbsp lemon juice
- ✓ 2 tbsp white wine vinegar
- ✓ Salt and black pepper, a generous pinch to your taste

DIRECTIONS:

- ➢ Mix together the salad ingredients in a large salad bowl
- ➢ In a separate smaller bowl or jar, mix together the dressing ingredients

- ➢ Drizzle the dressing over the salad and gently toss to coat
- ➢ Set aside for 30 minutes to allow the flavors to mix
- ➢ Serve and enjoy.

NUTRITION INFORMATION: Calories: 257; Carbs: 30.5g; Protein: 8.4g; Fats: 12.6g

194. BLUE CHEESE AND ARUGULA SALAD

Servings: 4   **Cook Time: 0 Min**   **Prep Time 10 Min**

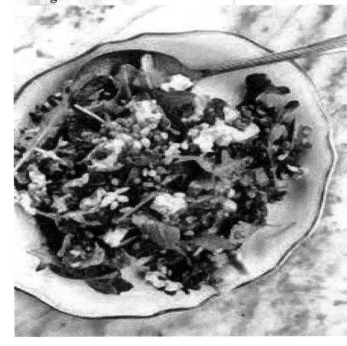

INGREDIENTS:

- ✓ ¼ cup crumbled blue cheese
- ✓ 1 tsp Dijon mustard
- ✓ 1-pint fresh figs, quartered
- ✓ 2 bags arugula
- ✓ 3 tbsp Balsamic Vinegar
- ✓ 3 tbsp olive oil
- ✓ Pepper and salt to taste

DIRECTIONS:

- ➢ Whisk thoroughly together pepper, salt, olive oil
- ➢ Dijon mustard, and balsamic vinegar to make the dressing
- ➢ Set aside in the ref for at least 30 minutes to marinate and allow the spices to combine
- ➢ On four serving plates, evenly arrange arugula
- ➢ Top with blue cheese and figs
- ➢ Drizzle each plate of salad with 1 ½ tbsp of prepared dressing
- ➢ Serve and enjoy.

NUTRITION INFORMATION: Calories: 202; Protein: 2.5g; Carbs: 25.5g; Fat: 10g

195. CHARRED TOMATO AND BROCCOLI SALAD

Servings: 6　　　　**Cook Time: 20 Min**　　　　**Prep Time 10 Min**

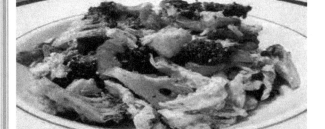

INGREDIENTS:
- ✓ ¼ cup lemon juice
- ✓ ½ tsp chili powder
- ✓ 1 ½ lbs. boneless chicken breast
- ✓ 1 ½ lbs. medium tomato
- ✓ 1 tsp freshly ground pepper
- ✓ 1 tsp salt
- ✓ 4 cups broccoli florets
- ✓ 5 tbsp extra virgin olive oil, divided to
- ✓ 2 and 3 tablespoons

DIRECTIONS:
➤ Place the chicken in a skillet and add just enough water to cover the chicken. Bring to a simmer over high heat
➤ Reduce the heat once the liquid boils and cook the chicken thoroughly for 12 minutes
➤ Once cooked, shred the chicken into bite-sized pieces
➤ On a large pot, bring water to a boil and add the broccoli
➤ Cook for 5 minutes until slightly tender
➤ Drain and rinse the broccoli with cold water. Set aside
➤ Core the tomatoes and cut them crosswise
➤ Discard the seeds and set the tomatoes cut side down on paper towels
➤ Pat them dry. In a heavy skillet, heat the pan over high heat until very hot
➤ Brush the cut sides of the tomatoes with olive oil and place them on the pan
➤ Cook the tomatoes until the sides are charred. Set aside
➤ In the same pan, heat the remaining 3 tablespoon olive oil over medium heat
➤ Stir the salt, chili powder and pepper and stir for 45 seconds
➤ Pour over the lemon juice and remove the pan from the heat
➤ Plate the broccoli, shredded chicken and chili powder mixture dressing.

NUTRITION INFORMATION: Calories: 210.8; Protein: 27.5g; Carbs: 6.3g; Fat: 8.4g

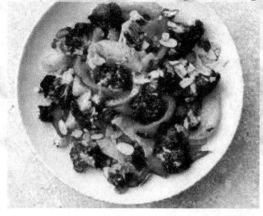

196. ALMOND-CRUSTED SWORDFISH

Servings: 4   **Cook Time: 15 Min**   **Prep Time 25 Min**

INGREDIENTS:

- ½ cup almond flour
- ¼ cup crushed Marcona almonds
- ½ to 1 teaspoon salt, divided
- 1 pounds (907 g) Swordfish, preferably
- 1 inch thick
- 1 large egg, beaten (optional)
- ¼ cup pure apple cider
- ¼ cup extra-virgin olive oil, plus more for frying
- 3 to 4 sprigs flat-leaf parsley, chopped
- 1 lemon, juiced
- 1 tablespoon Spanish paprika
- 5 medium baby portobello mushrooms, chopped (optional)
- 4 or 5 chopped scallions, both green and white parts
- 3 to 4 garlic cloves, peeled
- ¼ cup chopped pitted Kalamata olives

DIRECTIONS:

- On a dinner plate, spread the flour and crushed Marcona almonds and mix in the salt
- Alternately, pour the flour, almonds, and ¼ teaspoon of salt into a large plastic food storage bag
- Add the fish and coat it with the flour mixture
- If a thicker coat is desired, repeat this step after dipping the fish in the egg (if using).
- In a measuring cup, combine the apple cider, ¼ cup of olive oil
- Then parsley, lemon juice, paprika, and ¼ teaspoon of salt
- Mix well and set aside.
- In a large, heavy-bottom sauté pan or skillet
- Pour the olive oil to a depth of ⅛ inch and heat on medium heat
- Once the oil is hot, add the fish and brown for 3 to 5 minutes
- Then turn the fish over and add the mushrooms, scallions, garlic, and olives.
- Cook for an additional 3 minutes
- Once the other side of the fish is brown, remove the fish from the pan and set aside.
- Pour the cider mixture into the skillet and mix well with the vegetables
- Put the fried fish into the skillet on top of the mixture
- Cook with sauce on medium-low heat for 10 minutes
- (Until the fish flakes easily with a fork)
- Carefully remove the fish from the pan and plate
- Spoon the sauce over the fish
- Serve with white rice or home-fried potatoes.

NUTRITION INFORMATION: Calories: 620 fat: 37g protein: 63g carbs: 10g fiber: 5g sodium: 644mg

197. GREEK STYLE QUESADILLAS

Servings: 4   **Cook Time: 10 Min**   **Prep Time 10 Min**

INGREDIENTS:

- 4 whole wheat tortillas
- 1 cup Mozzarella cheese, shredded
- 1 cup fresh spinach, chopped
- 2 tablespoon Greek yogurt
- 1 egg, beaten
- 1/4 cup green olives, sliced
- 1 tablespoon olive oil
- 1/3 cup fresh cilantro, chopped

DIRECTIONS:

- In the bowl, combine together Mozzarella cheese, spinach, yogurt, egg, olives, and cilantro.
- Then pour olive oil in the skillet.
- In the skillet
- Place one tortilla and spread it with Mozzarella mixture.
- Top it with the second tortilla and spread it with cheese mixture again.
- Then place the third tortilla
- Spread it with all remaining cheese mixture.
- Cover it with the last tortilla
- Fry it for 5 minutes from each side over the medium heat.

NUTRITION INFORMATION: Calories: 193 Fat: 7.7g Fiber: 3.2g Carbs: 23.6g Protein: 8.3g

198. LIGHT PAPRIKA MOUSSAKA

Servings: 3   **Cook Time: 45 Min**   **Prep Time 15 Min**

INGREDIENTS:

- ✓ 1 eggplant, trimmed 1 cup ground chicken
- ✓ 1/3 cup white onion, diced
- ✓ 3 oz. Cheddar cheese, shredded
- ✓ 1 potato, sliced
- ✓ 1 teaspoon olive oil 1 teaspoon salt
- ✓ 1/2 cup milk
- ✓ 1 tablespoon butter
- ✓ 1 tablespoon ground paprika
- ✓ 1 tablespoon Italian seasoning
- ✓ 1 teaspoon tomato paste

DIRECTIONS:

- ➢ Slice the eggplant in length and sprinkle with salt.
- ➢ In the skillet Pour olive oil and add sliced potato.
- ➢ Roast potato for 2 minutes from each side.
- ➢ Then transfer it in the plate.
- ➢ Put eggplant in the skillet and roast it for 2 minutes from each side too.
- ➢ In the pan Pour milk and bring it to boil.
- ➢ Add tomato paste, Italian seasoning, paprika, butter, and Cheddar cheese.
- ➢ Then mix up together onion with ground chicken.
- ➢ Arrange the sliced potato in the casserole in one layer.
- ➢ Then add 1/2 part of all sliced eggplants.
- ➢ Spread the eggplants with 1/2 part of chicken mixture.
- ➢ Then add remaining eggplants.
- ➢ Pour the milk mixture over the eggplants.
- ➢ Bake moussaka for 30 minutes at 355F.

NUTRITION INFORMATION: Calories: 387 Fat: 21.2g Fiber: 8.9g Carbs: 26.3g Protein: 25.4g

199. CUCUMBER BOWL WITH SPICES AND GREEK YOGURT

Servings: 3   **Cook Time: 20 Min**   **Prep Time 10 Min**

INGREDIENTS:

- ✓ 4 cucumbers
- ✓ 1/2 teaspoon chili pepper
- ✓ 1/4 cup fresh parsley, chopped
- ✓ ¾ cup fresh dill, chopped
- ✓ 2 tablespoons lemon juice
- ✓ 1/2 teaspoon salt
- ✓ 1/2 teaspoon ground black pepper
- ✓ 1/4 teaspoon sage
- ✓ 1/2 teaspoon dried oregano
- ✓ 1/3 cup Greek yogurt

DIRECTIONS:

- ➢ Make the cucumber dressing: blend the dill and parsley until you get green mash.
- ➢ Then combine together green mash with lemon juice, salt
- ➢ Add ground black pepper, sage, dried oregano, Greek yogurt, and chili pepper.
- ➢ Churn the mixture well.
- ➢ Chop the cucumbers roughly
- ➢ Combine them with cucumber dressing. Mix up well.
- ➢ Refrigerate the cucumber for 20 minutes

NUTRITION INFORMATION: Calories: 114 Fat: 1.6g Fiber: 4.1g Carbs: 23.2g Protein: 7.6g

200. *TUNA POCKETS*

Servings: 4   **Cook Time: 20 Min**   **Prep Time 10 Min**

INGREDIENTS:

- ✓ 1 Whole wheat pitta bread
- ✓ 1 tbsp. olive oil
- ✓ 2 Lettuce leaves any variety
- ✓ ¼ Cucumber sliced

- ✓ 1 Medium tomato sliced
- ✓ 1 Small onion sliced
- ✓ ½ Can tuna chunks
- ✓ Salt to taste Pepper to taste

DIRECTIONS:

- ➤ In a small bowl break the tuna chunks, add olive oil
- ➤ Toast pitta bread and cut into 2.

- ➤ Open pitta bread and insert lettuce, tomato, cucumber
- ➤ Then and onion along with half the tuna.
- ➤ Sprinkle with salt and pepper if required.

NUTRITION INFORMATION: Calories: 193 Fat: 7.7g Fiber: 3.2g Carbs: 23.6g Protein: 8.3g

BUSY MAN DIET
INTRODUCTION

Our modern world, with all its wonders, has introduced clutter into our living and working habits, leading to a reduction in physical activity. Today, we spend most of our time commuting to work, sitting at our desks in the office or relaxing at home. Add to this the lack of time and you have the perfect way to gain weight and live an unbalanced life. After a long day at the airport and in rush hour traffic, a healthy meal is the last thing we need. We all do it the same way: we order food (we eat it after a long day) and we eat it in front of the TV. Politicians think that health is important and that we should give up certain things, and in some cases they are right: fast food, alcohol, fatty foods and sweets. It's a bit difficult, but it is difficult. It all comes down to the way food is prepared, the way food is made and changing your mindset.

RULES FOR HEALTHY EATING FOR BUSY PEOPLE

BLENDING EVERYTHING
Healthy eating for business - blending
There is a way to prepare healthy, nutritious corn in just a few minutes. Are you wondering how to do it? The answer is blending. Meal blended can replace brunch, lunch or dinner, or it can be a refreshing snack. You can use it to make meakes, soures or garlic sauces. What can be blended? All kinds of fruits, some, vegetables and everything else. Internet there are many bleriment recipes that are plenty and you can combine foood or experiment varieties that you like or love with food combinations. Smoothies are easier because of the low sugar content if you add some shortening or low-fat flavoured cream.

KEEP A GOOD SUPPLY
Often lunch breaks at work are spent to work instead of actually enjoying a meal. At these times we look for rastries, donuts or pizza tables. For example, I know the phone numbers of pizzerias and I know where to find pizzerias, and I order takeaways and order food that is unhealthy. This has to change. Find out which routes offer health information on Intélinet and the next time you want to order, choose them all. You will certainly notice how many spices and nutritional juices you can choose from! The seared chicken or the fried chicken, the vandalised chicken, the grilled chicken or the fried chicken, the fried chicken. You were hungry, right?

PROTEIN POWDERS AND BARS
Protein-rich foods have become essential for busssity lifestyles as there is less time to prepare food. When you're at work and waiting for work in the morning, going door-to-door. You're in the mood for a quick trip, and that's one of the things that briskets and bars come in handy for. In many cases, you may simply find that a flavour or granola bar is absolutely delicious to you and you want to incorporate it into your diet. Remember, however, that while these useful additions can be helpful ways to make you feel full, that doesn't mean they are essential in a rroper sense. It is recommended that you consume them regularly, but only as a supplement to a well-digested diet.

CARRY YOUR HEALTH IN BOTTLES

What is the first thing that comes to your mind when you think of healthy drink? If it's water, you're right. Your body needs water. Moisture in our bodies comes from fluids that are secreted through brushing, sweating and exercise. Water has an advantage: it is salty and contains no sugar

DO YOU WANT TO INCREASE YOUR PERFORMANCE AND EFFICIENCY?

Omega 3 is important for brain function and egg cell health, but our bodies don't produce it in significant quantities. Get this from the good Omega 3 Fish Oil Supplement. Always keep a small amount with you, in the car and at your desk. In this way, you can rejoice all the time. If you want to save money and avoid stopping when you realise you haven't bought anything in the evening, fill up the bottles. Use pitchers of the highest quality, and rour into bottle that you wilvers have before you leave the house. Watter filters reduce lead, zinc, copper, cadmium, mirsury, shromium, DDT and chlorine taste. If you like your wauce fizzy, you can add raw berries, raw berries, sliced and diced mochi or raw fruit.

PREPARED FOR WORKWEEK ACCORDINGLY.

Healthy eating for businesses - Soontainers

Food preparation is important for maintaining a healthy diet and losing or gaining weight. When healthy meals are inexpensive, we are more inclined to order them from fast food restaurants rather than simply fast food or stopping. Also, by doing so, we reduce the streess and anxiety of trying to figure out what to eat each day for our lives. The key is preparation. It simple - it's about having ready-made recipes that you can use and enjoy throughout the weekend. Plus, it all happens in one day, so you don't have to stress about it all day long.

BE CAREFUL WHAT YOU ORDER IN RESTAURANTS

Sometimes people go to restaurants believing that this will improve their health, but they don't have to if they have eaten, enjoyed and consumed their meals carefully to keep fit. Even if you eat out at a restaurant or diner, you have the health information to make sure your taste buds are healthy. If you don't want to eat more than you would when you serve your own food, be aware of when, where and what you eat - don't clean your plate! Try to eat lunch, take your time and eat when you are full.

ENJOY FRUIT AND VEGETABLES EVERYWHERE.

Fruits and vegetables are rich in vitamins, antioxidants and minerals. They also reduce the risk of Type 2 diabetes, strock, cardiovascular disease and even illness. Maternity drums can make life light and flawless because they are light, light and light. A fruitful and healthy diet contributes to weight loss or maintaining a healthy lifestyle.

HIDDEN INFLAMMATION INSIDE YOUR BODY PERHAPS CAUSING YOUR TIREDNESS

Turmeric may be just what you need to relieve inflammation and restore energy. Make sure you meet your daily requirement of fresh foods, as well as fresh snacks, to make hunger go away. Trick is to leave fruits and vegetables in places tactical. Leave an apple on your desk and a bernard in a box. No oranges in the car; i.e. - in the glove compartment. Put a cricket on the living room table and maybe some grapes. Of course, it's up to you and your fruit and vegetables.

CHOOSE YOUR YOGHURT

Yoghurt can be a good addition to a healthy diet, but like any other food, it should be prepared in a varied and diverse way. It is a great dary product, rich in salsium and protein, but also in fat and sallories. Finding a diet that meets your needs is important, and is determined by how much you eat per day, as many are more nutritionally sound than others. For example, if you don't want to use low-fat urea cheese, which is very nutritious, you can add other foods, such as fruit for a sweeter taste or nuts, which add nutritional value and provide a nutritious and healthy diet.

HEALTHY SANDWICH OPTIONS WORTHY OF A KING

Worry-free design and prepared with a variety of nutrients - the sandwich is the perfect shoice, combining whole grains, vegetables and protein into one delicious bite. Basically, it's two rieces of bread, with a room in between - and it has a lot of taced nutrients, and if done right, it's a great and healthy option. So, if you want to do something right, do it yourself. If you want to make a low-calorie sandwich without sacrificing good taste or satisfaction try adding some avocados or cucumber, pile with veggies, choose whole-gran and skip bread altogether. Try introduce some meatless proteins or simply think out basic of meat and sheese and add flavor with low-calorie toppings. And at the end of the day, reastion - it's not just about losing weight, it's about keeping fit.

201. *THAI STEAMED SALMON*

Servings: 2　　　　　　**Cook Time: 20 Min**　　　　　　**Prep Time 10 Min**

INGREDIENTS:

- 1 bunch coriander, washed
- 12 mint leaves
- 1 tsp chopped fresh ginger
- 3 cloves garlic, crushed
- 1 tsp salt

TO SERVE

- Basmati rice, washed in cold water until the water runs clear
- 1 chilli, finely sliced

- 1 large red chilli, finely chopped
- juice of 2 limes
- 1 tbsp nam pla (fish sauce)
- 2 x 175g/6oz salmon fillets
- 4 bok choi, cut in half lengthways

- Bunch coriander, roughly chopped
- Pinch salt
- 1 lime, cut into wedges

DIRECTIONS:

- In a food processor blend together the coriander leaves
- Then stalks, the mint leaves, ginger, garlic, salt, chilli, lime juice and fish sauce and process until smooth.
- Place the salmon fillets in a shallow dish
- Pour over half of the sauce. Leave to marinate for 20 minutes.
- Pour the rice into a pan of boiling water
- Cook according to the packet instructions.
- Turn on the steamer and place the bok choi on the bottom layer

- Place the marinated salmon fillets in the top half of the steamer
- Cook for 6- 8 minutes until the fish is just cooked and the bok choi is tender.
- Drain the rice and stir through the sliced chilli and roughly chopped coriander
- Season with salt and divide between serving plates.
- Remove the salmon and bok choi from the steamer
- Arrange on top of the rice
- Pour the reserved sauce over the salmon and serve immediately with a wedge of lime.

Servings: 6   **Cook Time: 1 H**   **Prep Time 10 Min**

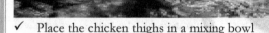

INGREDIENTS:

- ✓ 8 chicken thighs, bone-in, skin removed
- ✓ 150ml/¼ pint dark soy sauce
- ✓ 4 tbsp sherry or cider vinegar
- ✓ 2 tbsp light olive oil
- ✓ 1 tbsp coarsely ground black pepper
- ✓ 2 tbsp finely grated ginger
- ✓ 2 tbsp finely grated garlic
- ✓ 2 bay leaves
- ✓ 2 large carrots, cut into bite-sized cubes
- ✓ 400ml/14fl oz chicken stock
- ✓ 200g/7oz brown basmati rice
- ✓ 1 tbsp cornflour
- ✓ 8 spring onions, finely sliced

DIRECTIONS:

- ✓ Place the chicken thighs in a mixing bowl
- ✓ Mix together the soy sauce, vinegar, 1 tablespoon of the oil, the coarsely ground pepper
- ✓ Add half of the grated ginger and half of the grated garlic
- ✓ Pour this over the chicken and toss to coat well
- ✓ Cover and marinate in the fridge for 1 hour.
- ✓ Heat the remaining oil in a wide, non-stick frying pan (that has a lid)
- ✓ Remove the chicken from the marinade (reserving the marinade)
- ✓ Brown the chicken for 3–4 minutes on each side
- ✓ Transfer to a plate and set aside.
- ✓ Return the pan to the heat and add the remaining oil, garlic and ginger and stir-fry for 1 minute
- ✓ Return the chicken to the pan with the reserved marinade, bay leaves, carrots and stock.
- ✓ Bring to a boil, reduce the heat to low and allow to simmer for 40 minutes
- ✓ Cover the pan with the lid for the last 15 minutes, or until the chicken is cooked through.
- ✓ Meanwhile, cook the rice according to the packet instructions and keep warm.
- ✓ In a small bowl, mix the cornflour with 2 tablespoons cold water until smooth
- ✓ Stir the cornflour mixture through the chicken and sauce
- ✓ Cook for another 4–5 minutes, or until the sauce has thickened.
- ✓ Remove from the heat, sprinkle over the spring onions
- ✓ Serve with the brown rice.

203. WARM CHICKEN SALAD

Servings: 6　　　　**Cook Time: 1 H**　　　　**Prep Time 10 Min**

INGREDIENTS:

- ✓ 2 small chicken breasts, boned, skinned and cut in half
- ✓ calorie controlled cooking oil spray
- ✓ 1 large orange or red pepper, deseeded and cut in to chunks
- ✓ 1 little gem lettuce, leaves separated
- ✓ 50g/1¾oz watercress, tough stalks removed
- ✓ 2 ripe medium tomatoes, cut into small chunks
- ✓ ⅓ cucumber, sliced
- ✓ 1 tsp thick balsamic vinegar
- ✓ ½ small lemon, juice only
- ✓ Sea salt and freshly ground black pepper

DIRECTIONS:

- ➢ Season the chicken pieces on both sides with salt and pepper
- ➢ Spray a large non-stick frying pan with oil and place over a high heat
- ➢ Cook the chicken pieces for three minutes on each side
- ➢ (Or until lightly browned and cooked through)
- ➢ Transfer to a plate.
- ➢ Spray the pan with a little more oil
- ➢ Cook the pepper for three minutes on each side
- ➢ (Or until lightly charred and beginning to soften)
- ➢ Arrange the lettuce leaves, watercress, tomatoes, cucumber and pepper on two plates.
- ➢ Slice the chicken breasts and scatter on top of salad
- ➢ Drizzle with the balsamic vinegar and squeeze the lemon juice over
- ➢ Season with black pepper and serve.

204. CHICKEN AND LEEK TRAYBAKE

Servings: 4　　　　**Cook Time: 50 Min**　　　　**Prep Time 10 Min**

INGREDIENTS:

- ✓ 2 leeks, halved and finely sliced
- ✓ 6 fresh thyme sprigs
- ✓ 4 garlic cloves, crushed
- ✓ 2 x 250g packet vacuum-packed puy lentils
- ✓ 200g/7oz radishes, halved
- ✓ 4 free-range chicken breasts
- ✓ 4 tsp mustard
- ✓ 40g/1½oz panko breadcrumbs
- ✓ 20g/¾oz fresh flat-leaf parsley, finely chopped
- ✓ 1½ tbsp olive oil
- ✓ 300ml/10fl oz hot chicken stock
- ✓ 4 tbsp crème fraîche
- ✓ Sea salt and freshly ground black pepper

DIRECTIONS:

- ➢ Preheat the oven to 200C/180C Fan/Gas 6.
- ➢ Place the leek, thyme, garlic, lentils and radishes in a roasting tin
- ➢ Stir to combine and make four indentations in the mixture
- ➢ Place the chicken breasts in the indentations
- ➢ Cover each breast with a teaspoon of mustard.
- ➢ Mix together the breadcrumbs, parsley, olive oil and sea salt in a small bowl
- ➢ Scatter evenly over the mustard on each chicken breast.
- ➢ Carefully pour the stock into the tin
- ➢ Cover the vegetables and around the chicken breasts
- ➢ Take care not to get any stock on the breadcrumbs.
- ➢ Roast for 35–40 minutes, or until the chicken is cooked through and the breadcrumbs are crisp and golden
- ➢ The chicken is cooked when the juices run clear
- ➢ (With no trace of pink when the thickest part of the breast is pierced with a skewer)
- ➢ Leave the dish to stand for 10 minutes.
- ➢ Stir in crème fraîche and season with salt and pepper. Serve immediately.

205. CHICKEN AND TARRAGON OMELETTE

Servings: 2   **Cook Time: 20 Min**   **Prep Time 10 Min**

INGREDIENTS:
- ✓ 1 leek, thinly sliced
- ✓ 2 tbsp vegetable or chicken stock
- ✓ 4 tbsp fat-free quark or fat-free natural cottage cheese
- ✓ 1 tbsp finely chopped fresh tarragon
- ✓ 1 cooked chicken breast, skin removed, cut into small dice
- ✓ Llow-calorie cooking spray
- ✓ 4 large free-range eggs, beaten
- ✓ Salt and freshly ground black pepper

TO SERVE (OPTIONAL)
- ✓ 4 plum tomatoes, halved
- ✓ ½ cucumber, finely chopped

DIRECTIONS:
- ➤ Preheat the oven to 120C/100C Fan/Gas ¼ .
- ➤ Put the leeks and stock in a small saucepan and cover
- ➤ Cook for 5–6 minutes, or until tender and all the liquids have been absorbed
- ➤ Season and stir in the quark, tarragon and chicken.
- ➤ Spray a 20cm/8in frying pan with low-calorie cooking spray
- ➤ Place over a high heat.
- ➤ Season the eggs, then add half to the pan
- ➤ Cook, pushing the cooked egg into the centre of the pan
- ➤ Allow the runny egg to flow into its place until no runny egg is left.
- ➤ Spoon half the chicken mixture into the middle of the omelette
- ➤ Flip one side on top of the chicken
- ➤ Then the other side over to encase the filling
- ➤ Roll the omelette onto a plate and keep warm while you cook the second one.
- ➤ Meanwhile, toss together the tomatoes and cucumber
- ➤ Serve the omelettes with the cucumber salad.

206. CHICKEN AND VEGETABLE BALTI

Servings: 4   **Cook Time: 40 Min**   **Prep Time 10 Min**

INGREDIENTS:

- ✓ Calorie controlled cooking oil spray
- ✓ 1 medium onion, thinly sliced
- ✓ 4 chicken thighs, boned and skinned
- ✓ 1 red pepper, deseeded and cut into 3cm/1in chunks
- ✓ 1 yellow pepper, deseeded and cut into 3cm/1in chunks
- ✓ 1 tbsp cornflour

- ✓ 150g/5½oz fat-free natural yogurt
- ✓ 1 tbsp medium or mild curry powder
- ✓ 2 garlic cloves, thinly sliced
- ✓ 227g/8oz tin chopped tomatoes
- ✓ 3 heaped tbsp finely chopped fresh coriander, plus extra to garnish
- ✓ Freshly ground black pepper

DIRECTIONS:

- ➢ Spray a large, deep, non-stick frying pan or wok with oil and place over a medium heat
- ➢ Add the onion and cook for five minutes, stirring regularly until well softened and lightly browned.
- ➢ Meanwhile, trim all the visible fat off the chicken thighs
- ➢ Cut each one into four pieces and season with black pepper.
- ➢ Then the chicken and peppers into the pan with the onion
- ➢ Cook for three minutes, turning occasionally.
- ➢ Meanwhile, in a small bowl, mix the cornflour with 2 tablespoons cold water

- ➢ Stir in the yoghurt until thoroughly mixed.
- ➢ Sprinkle the curry powder over the chicken and vegetables
- ➢ Add the garlic and cook for 30 seconds.
- ➢ Tip the tomatoes into the pan, add the yoghurt mixture, 150ml/3½fl oz of water and coriander.
- ➢ Bring to a gentle simmer and cook for 20-25 minutes
- ➢ Stir occasionally until the chicken is tender and the sauce is thick
- ➢ Season with freshly ground black pepper to taste and garnish with coriander.

207. CHICKEN AND CASHEW NOODLE STIR-FRY

Servings: 4   **Cook Time: 40 Min**   **Prep Time 10 Min**

INGREDIENTS:

- ✓ 1 tbsp vegetable oil
- ✓ 250g/9oz chicken breast, cut into thin strips
- ✓ 1 tbsp runny honey
- ✓ 1 garlic clove, crushed
- ✓ 1 tbsp chopped fresh ginger
- ✓ ½ red chilli, finely chopped
- ✓ 3 spring onions, chopped
- ✓ 1 small carrot, sliced

- ✓ 1 red pepper, cut into strips
- ✓ 1 head of pak choi, chopped
- ✓ 300g/10½oz straight-to-wok fine egg noodles
- ✓ Small bunch fresh coriander, roughly chopped
- ✓ 1 tbsp dark soy sauce
- ✓ 1 tbsp toasted sesame oil
- ✓ 1 lime, finely grated zest and juice
- ✓ 25g/1oz unsalted, toasted cashew nuts

DIRECTIONS:

- ➢ Heat a large wok over a high heat. Add half the oil and the chicken
- ➢ Stir fry for 1 minute, then add the honey and fry until the chicken is fully cooked and a rich golden-brown
- ➢ Remove from the wok and set aside.
- ➢ Add the remaining oil to the wok and fry the garlic, ginger and chilli for 20 seconds over a medium heat

- ➢ Then the vegetables and stir-fry until they are just tender but retain some bite
- ➢ Add the pre-cooked noodles and sauté for a minute or so before returning the chicken to the pan.
- ➢ Join also the coriander, soy sauce, sesame oil and lime zest and juice and toss well.
- ➢ Serve with a scattering of cashews over the top.

208. CHICKEN NOODLE SALAD

Servings: 2   **Cook Time: 20 Min**   **Prep Time 10 Min**

INGREDIENTS:

- ✓ 70g/2½oz medium egg noodles
- ✓ 50g/1¾oz frozen soya beans or frozen peas
- ✓ 1 carrot, peeled
- ✓ ½ small red pepper, seeds removed, sliced
- ✓ 75g/2¾oz mangetout, trimmed and halved lengthways
- ✓ 1 cooked boneless, skinless chicken breast (about 125g/4½oz)
- ✓ 4 spring onions, trimmed and finely sliced
- ✓ 1 long red chilli, finely sliced (deseeded if preferred)
- ✓ 15g/½oz fresh coriander leaves
- ✓ 10g/⅓oz fresh mint leaves
- ✓ 15g/½oz roasted cashew nuts, roughly chopped

- ✓ 4 tsp dark soy sauce
- ✓ 1 tsp toasted sesame oil

FOR THE DRESSING

- ✓ 3 tbsp water
- ✓ 3 tsp caster sugar
- ✓ ½–1 tsp dried chilli flakes, to taste

DIRECTIONS:

- ➤ To make the dressing, place the water, sugar and chilli flakes in a small saucepan over a low heat and warm gently
- ➤ (Until the sugar is dissolved)
- ➤ Bring to the boil and cook for 30 seconds, stirring
- ➤ Take off the heat and stir in the soy sauce and sesame oil. Leave to cool.
- ➤ Half-fill a saucepan with water
- ➤ Bring to the boil. Add the noodles
- ➤ Cook for 3–4 minutes, or according to the packet instructions, until tender. Stir occasionally to separate the strands
- ➤ Add the soya beans or peas to the noodles
- ➤ Stir well and then immediately drain in a colander

- ➤ Rinse the noodles and beans under cold running water
- ➤ (Until the mixture is completely cool)
- ➤ Tip into a large mixing bowl.
- ➤ Carefully peel the carrot into long, wide ribbons or cut into long, thin matchsticks
- ➤ Add the carrot, pepper and mangetout to the noodle salad
- ➤ Cut the chicken into thin slices and place in the bowl.
- ➤ Pour the dressing into the bowl and toss so everything is well mixed
- ➤ Add the spring onions, red chilli, fresh herbs and nuts to the bowl
- ➤ Toss lightly before serving.

Servings: 4   **Cook Time: 40 Min**   **Prep Time 10 Min**

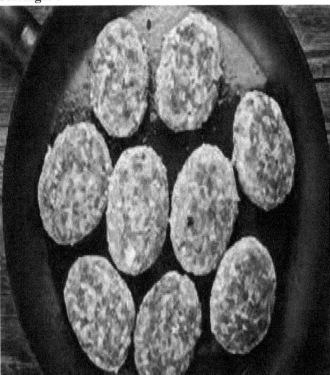

INGREDIENTS:
- ✓ 250g/9oz chana dal, soaked overnight or for at least 2 hours
- ✓ 1 garlic clove
- ✓ 1 tsp red chilli powder
- ✓ ½ tsp ground turmeric
- ✓ 1 cinnamon stick
- ✓ 1 onion, thinly sliced
- ✓ 1–2 tbsp ghee
- ✓ Salt, to taste

FOR THE TARKA
- ✓ 1–2 tbsp ghee
- ✓ 2 garlic cloves, thinly sliced
- ✓ 1 tsp cumin seeds
- ✓ 1 tsp mustard seeds
- ✓ 2 long dried red chillies
- ✓ 5–6 curry leaves (fresh if possible)

TO SERVE
- ✓ 2 tbsp tamarind chutney (available in Asian shops)
- ✓ 2.5cm/1in piece root ginger, peeled and very thinly sliced
- ✓ Handful mixed fresh coriander, dill and chervil, finely chopped
- ✓ 1 tsp chaat masala

DIRECTIONS:
- ➢ Drain the chana dal and put it into a large saucepan with the garlic, red chilli powder, turmeric, cinnamon stick and salt.
- ➢ Pour in 350ml/12fl oz water, or enough to cover the dal and bring it to the boil.
- ➢ Cook for 15–20 minutes, or until soft
- ➢ Look for a firm and not mushy dal
- ➢ If it is a little watery, using a wooden spoon
- ➢ Crush some lentils around the sides of the pan to thicken the sauce
- ➢ Season the dal and put it in a serving bowl.
- ➢ Meanwhile, fry the onion in the ghee until browned
- ➢ Then transfer it to kitchen paper and set aside.
- ➢ For the tarka, melt the ghee in a small frying pan over a medium heat
- ➢ Fry the garlic until it starts to brown lightly
- ➢ Add the cumin and mustard seeds and cook until they splutter
- ➢ Quickly add the dried red chillies and curry leaves and cook for 5 seconds
- ➢ Immediately pour the tarka over the dal.
- ➢ Garnish with the tamarind chutney, onions, herbs, ginger and chaat masala.

210.   *SLOW COOKER LAMB AND SWEET POTATO TAGINE*

Servings: 4   **Cook Time: 6-10 H**   **Prep Time 10 Min**

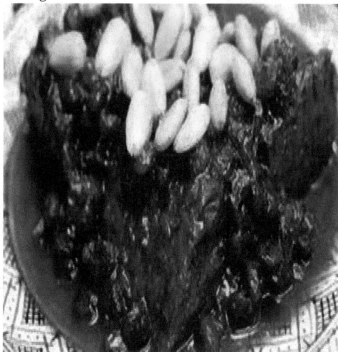

INGREDIENTS:
FOR THE TAGINE
- ✓ 600g/1lb 5oz lamb neck fillet, trimmed of any excess fat and cut into 3cm chunks
- ✓ 2 tbsp harissa paste
- ✓ 3 garlic cloves, finely chopped or grated
- ✓ 1 tsp ground cumin
- ✓ 1 tsp ground coriander
- ✓ 1 tsp ground cinnamon
- ✓ 1 tsp smoked paprika
- ✓ 1 onion, roughly chopped
- ✓ 90g/3¼oz dried apricots, roughly chopped
- ✓ 90g/3¼oz drained pitted green olives
- ✓ 1 x 400g tin chopped tomatoes
- ✓ 1 x 400g tin chickpeas, drained and rinsed
- ✓ 500g/1lb 2oz sweet potatoes, peeled and cut into chunks
- ✓ 350ml/12fl oz chicken stock, from a cube
- ✓ 90g/3¼oz low-fat plain yoghurt
- ✓ 1 small bunch coriander, roughly chopped
- ✓ ½ tsp sea salt
- ✓ Freshly ground black pepper

- ✓ ½ chicken stock cube
- ✓ 250g/9oz cherry tomatoes, halved, quartered if large
- ✓ 1 small bunch mint, leaves picked and roughly chopped

FOR THE COUSCOUS
- ✓ 200g/7oz couscous
- ✓ 1 lemon, zest and juice
- ✓ 1 tsp ground cumin
- ✓ 1 tsp sweet smoked paprika
- ✓ 1 red onion, finely chopped
- ✓ 2 green peppers, deseeded and roughly chopped

DIRECTIONS:
- ➤ Preheat the slow cooker on the high setting.
- ➤ Put the lamb into the slow cooker
- ➤ Add the harissa paste, garlic, spices, salt and pepper and mix well
- ➤ Then the onions and apricots, olives, chopped tomatoes, chickpeas, sweet potato and chicken stock
- ➤ Stir well and cover with the lid.
- ➤ Leave the tagine to cook on high for 6–8 hours, or on low for 8–10 hours.
- ➤ Put the couscous into a large bowl

- ➤ Add the lemon zest and juice, ground cumin, smoked paprika, onion and peppers and stir well
- ➤ Join also the chicken stock cube and pour over 250ml/9fl oz boiling water
- ➤ Cover with cling film and leave for 10 minutes.
- ➤ Use a fork to fluff up the couscous
- ➤ Then stir through the cherry tomatoes and mint.
- ➤ Serve the tagine with the couscous
- ➤ Top with a dollop of yoghurt and finish with a scatter of chopped coriander.

211. EASY VEGETABLE STIR- FRY

Servings: 2 **Cook Time: 15 Min** **Prep Time 10 Min**

INGREDIENTS:

- ✓ 2 tbsp sunflower oil
- ✓ 4 spring onions, cut into 4cm/1½in lengths
- ✓ 1 garlic clove, crushed
- ✓ Piece fresh root ginger, about 1cm/½in, peeled and grated
- ✓ 1 carrot, cut into matchsticks
- ✓ 1 red pepper, cut into thick matchsticks
- ✓ 100g/3½oz baby sweetcorn, halved
- ✓ 1 courgette, cut into thick matchsticks
- ✓ 150g/5½oz sugar-snap peas or mangetout, trimmed
- ✓ 2 tbsp hoisin sauce
- ✓ 2 tbsp low-salt soy sauce

DIRECTIONS:

- ➢ Heat a wok on a high heat and add the sunflower oil
- ➢ Add the spring onions, garlic, ginger and stir-fry for 1 minute
- ➢ Then reduce the heat. Take care to not brown the vegetables.
- ➢ Add the carrot, red pepper and baby sweetcorn and stir-fry for 2 minutes
- ➢ Add the courgette and sugar snap peas and stir-fry for a further 3 minutes
- ➢ Toss the ingredients from the centre to the side of the wok using a wooden spatula
- ➢ Do not overcrowd the wok and keep the ingredients moving.
- ➢ Then 1 tablespoon water, hoisin and soy sauce
- ➢ Cook over a high heat for a further 2 minutes
- ➢ (Or until all the vegetables are cooked but not too soft)
- ➢ Serve with noodles or rice.

212. RAINBOW NOODLES

Servings: 2 **Cook Time: 15 Min** **Prep Time 10 Min**

INGREDIENTS:

- ✓ 250g/9oz wholewheat egg noodles
- ✓ 1 tbsp vegetable oil
- ✓ 1 red pepper, seeds removed and finely sliced
- ✓ 1 small bunch spring onions, finely sliced
- ✓ 2 garlic cloves, finely chopped
- ✓ 2 large carrots, peeled into ribbons with vegetable peeler
- ✓ 1 medium courgette, peeled into ribbons with a vegetable peeler, then shredded
- ✓ 3 tbsp soy sauce
- ✓ 2 tbsp sweet chilli sauce
- ✓ 1 lime, juice only
- ✓ 150ml/5fl oz vegetable stock
- ✓ 25g/1oz roasted unsalted peanuts, lightly crushed
- ✓ 2 tbsp roughly chopped fresh coriander
- ✓ 1 red chilli, roughly chopped

DIRECTIONS:

- ➢ Bring a large saucepan of water to the boil
- ➢ Cook the noodles according to packet instructions. Drain and set aside.
- ➢ Heat the oil in a wok over a high heat and stir-fry the pepper for 2 minutes, until just softened
- ➢ Add the spring onion and garlic and stir-fry for another minute
- ➢ Then the carrot and courgette and stir-fry for 1 minute.
- ➢ Put the soy, sweet chilli sauce, lime juice
- ➢ Stock into a jam jar, screw the lid on and shake until combined.
- ➢ Pour the dressing into the wok
- ➢ Bring to the boil, simmer for 1 minute until the vegetables have softened.
- ➢ Stir in the drained noodles and heat through
- ➢ Top with the crushed peanuts, chopped coriander and chilli. Serve.

213. VERSATILE VEGETABLE STEW

Servings: 2 **Cook Time: 25 Min** **Prep Time 10 Min**

INGREDIENTS:

- ✓ 1 tbsp olive oil
- ✓ 1 onion, finely diced
- ✓ 2 leeks, split lengthways up to the root several times, washed under running cold water then sliced thickly
- ✓ 2 carrots, cut into 1cm/½in dice
- ✓ 2 garlic cloves, finely diced
- ✓ 1 tsp sweet smoked paprika
- ✓ ½ tsp dried thyme

- ✓ 2 potatoes, peeled, cut into 1cm/½in dice
- ✓ 600ml/21fl oz vegetable stock
- ✓ ½ head cauliflower, cut into small florets
- ✓ 200g/7oz fine green beans, cut into 2cm/¾in pieces
- ✓ 1 x 400g/14oz tin baked beans
- ✓ 2 tbsp roughly chopped flatleaf parsley
- ✓ Crusty bread, to serve
- ✓ Salt and freshly ground black pepper

DIRECTIONS:

- ➤ Heat a large frying pan or saucepan until medium hot, add the olive oil, onion
- ➤ Add leeks and cook gently for 5 minutes until just softened.
- ➤ Then the carrots, garlic, paprika and thyme and stir to combine
- ➤ Cook for 5 minutes.
- ➤ Add the potatoes and vegetable stock
- ➤ Bring to the boil. Turn the heat down and simmer for 5 minutes

- ➤ (Until the potatoes are just softening)
- ➤ Then add the cauliflower and simmer for another 5 minutes.
- ➤ By now, all the vegetables should be nearly cooked
- ➤ Add the green beans and baked beans
- ➤ Cook for 3 minutes then stir in the chopped parsley
- ➤ Season well with salt and pepper.
- ➤ Serve with plenty of crusty bread.

214. CHORIZO AND BUTTERBEAN STEW WITH BAKED POTATOES

Servings: 4 **Cook Time: 40 Min** **Prep Time 10 Min**

INGREDIENTS:

- ✓ 4 baking potatoes (200g/7oz each)
- ✓ 200g/7oz cooking chorizo, sliced
- ✓ 2 x 400g tins chopped tomatoes with onion and garlic

- ✓ 2 x 400g tins butter beans, drained
- ✓ 50g/1¾oz fresh basil leaves, roughly chopped
- ✓ Salt and freshly ground black pepper

DIRECTIONS:

- ➤ Preheat the oven to 220C/200C Fan/Gas 7.
- ➤ Prick the potatoes all over with a fork and microwave on a high heat for 5– 6 minutes
- ➤ Season well with salt
- ➤ Bake for 10–15 minutes, or until tender
- ➤ (If you don't have a microwave, bake for 1 hour at 220C/200C Fan/Gas 7).
- ➤ Meanwhile, dry-fry the chorizo in a large saucepan over a medium heat

- ➤ (For 4–5 minutes, or until lightly browned)
- ➤ Stir in the chopped tomatoes and beans and bring to a boil
- ➤ Reduce the heat to medium
- ➤ Cook for 12–15 minutes until slightly thickened, stirring often
- ➤ Season and stir in the basil.
- ➤ Serve the stew with the baked potatoes

215. PRAWN AND TOMATO PASTA

Servings: 2   **Cook Time: 20 Min**   **Prep Time 10 Min**

INGREDIENTS:

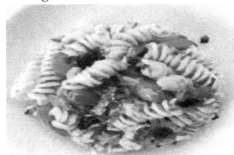

- ✓ 125g/4½oz dried spaghetti or linguine
- ✓ 150g/5½oz broccoli, cut into small florets
- ✓ 100g/3½oz cherry tomatoes, halved
- ✓ 150g/5½oz large frozen prawns, completely thawed and drained
- ✓ 1 tbsp extra virgin olive oil
- ✓ ½ tsp dried chilli flakes, to taste
- ✓ Sea salt and freshly ground black pepper
- ✓ Lemon wedges, for squeezing (optional)

DIRECTIONS:

- ➢ Half-fill a large, non-stick saucepan with water
- ➢ Bring to the boil. Add the pasta to the boiling water
- ➢ Return to the boil and cook for 8 minutes, stirring occasionally
- ➢ Add the broccoli to the pan and cook for 2 minutes more.
- ➢ Drain the pasta and broccoli

- ➢ Return to the pan and add the tomatoes, prawns, oil, chilli flakes and season well
- ➢ Cook for 2–3 minutes, tossing with two wooden spoons
- ➢ (Until the spaghetti is evenly coated with the spices from the pan and the prawns and tomatoes are hot)
- ➢ Squeeze over a little lemon juice, if using, and serve immediately

216. SPICY AUTUMN SQUASH STEW

Servings: 4   **Cook Time: 30 Min**   **Prep Time 10 Min**

INGREDIENTS:

- ✓ 2 tbsp sunflower oil
- ✓ 1 onion, finely chopped
- ✓ 2 garlic cloves, finely chopped
- ✓ 1 small red chilli, very finely chopped (or dried red chilli flakes, to taste)
- ✓ 1 red pepper, cut into short strips
- ✓ 6 spring onions, sliced diagonally
- ✓ 1 tsp ground coriander

- ✓ 1 medium butternut squash, peeled, deseeded, and rough cut into 2cm/1in pieces
- ✓ 2 handfuls cherry tomatoes, halved
- ✓ 400ml tin coconut milk
- ✓ ½ lemon, juice only
- ✓ Salt and freshly ground black pepper
- ✓ Small bunch coriander, leaves and stalks chopped separately

DIRECTIONS:

- ➢ Heat the oil in a a heavy-bottomed saucepan
- ➢ Add the onion, garlic, chilli, red pepper and spring onions
- ➢ Cook gently for about 5 minutes until soft.
- ➢ Add the ground coriander and cook for a minute
- ➢ Then add the squash, coriander stalks, and tomatoes
- ➢ Cook this for a further 5 minutes.

- ➢ Add the coconut milk and simmer, partially covered, for 15 minutes
- ➢ (Or until the squash is tender)
- ➢ Add the lemon juice
- ➢ Season with salt and freshly ground black pepper to taste
- ➢ Sprinkle over the coriander leaves
- ➢ Serve with white or brown basmati rice.

217. SPAGHETTI WITH ROASTED RIB RAGU

Servings: 4　　　　　**Cook Time: 1H 10 Min**　　　　　**Prep Time 10 Min**

INGREDIENTS:
- ✓ 3 tbsp olive oil
- ✓ 2 beef short ribs
- ✓ 1 red onion, quartered
- ✓ 1 yellow onion, quartered
- ✓ 2 large carrots, cut into 4cm/2in batons
- ✓ 15 tomatoes, preferably heritage tomatoes of assorted colours
- ✓ 1 garlic bulb
- ✓ 500ml/18fl oz beef stock
- ✓ 500g/1lb 2oz dried spaghetti
- ✓ Salt and freshly ground black pepper

DIRECTIONS:
- ➤ Preheat the oven to 180C/160 fan/Gas 4.
- ➤ Heat the oil over a medium heat in a large roasting tin on the hob
- ➤ Add the short ribs and fry for 3-4 minutes on all sides, or until browned all over
- ➤ Then the onions and carrots, then transfer to the oven for 45 minutes.
- ➤ After 45 minutes, tuck the tomatoes
- ➤ Add the whole garlic bulb into the roasting tin, pour in the beef stock and continue to cook for a further hour.
- ➤ Towards the end of the cooking time
- ➤ Cook the spaghetti according to the packet instructions, then drain well and set aside.
- ➤ Remove the beef ribs from the roasting tin and set aside on a chopping board to rest.
- ➤ Squeeze the garlic cloves from their skins into the roasting tin
- ➤ Using a slotted spoon or fork, lightly squash the tomatoes
- ➤ Mix them and the garlic into the sauce.
- ➤ Slide the short-rib meat off the bones and cut it into strips
- ➤ Return the meat to the roasting tin.
- ➤ Stir in the cooked pasta
- ➤ Then season with salt and freshly ground black pepper, and serve.

218. PENNE WITH ROASTED VEGETABLE AND TOMATO SAUCE

Servings: 4　　　　　**Cook Time: 30 Min**　　　　　**Prep Time 10 Min**

INGREDIENTS:
- ✓ 300g/10½oz penne
- ✓ 400g tin chopped tomatoes
- ✓ 2 tbsp extra virgin olive oil
- ✓ Pinch onion powder
- ✓ Pinch garlic granules
- ✓ ½ tsp chipotle sauce, or to taste
- ✓ 250g/9oz frozen roasted Mediterranean vegetables
- ✓ Salt and freshly ground black pepper
- ✓ 4 tbsp freshly grated Parmesan (or vegetarian alternative), to serve

DIRECTIONS:
- ➤ Bring a large saucepan of salted water to the boil
- ➤ Add the penne and cook according to the packet instructions, normally 10–12 minutes.
- ➤ Meanwhile, tip the tomatoes into a large saucepan
- ➤ Add the oil, onion powder, garlic granules and chipotle sauce
- ➤ Stir well, then bring to the boil over a medium heat. Simmer for 2 minutes.
- ➤ Remove from the heat and blend until smooth using a stick blender
- ➤ Return to the heat, stir in the roasted vegetables
- ➤ Cook for 2–3 minutes, or until bubbling.
- ➤ Drain the penne, reserving a little of the water
- ➤ Then tip the pasta into the sauce and stir
- ➤ Join also a couple of spoonfuls of pasta water to the pan
- ➤ Then season well with black pepper.
- ➤ Serve sprinkled with grated Parmesan or vegetarian alternative to serve.

219. *VEGETABLE CURRY*

Servings: 2 | **Cook Time: 30 Min** | **Prep Time 10 Min**

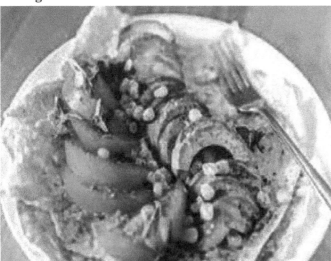

INGREDIENTS:

- ✓ 2 medium potatoes (around 350g/12oz), peeled and cut into 2cm chunks
- ✓ 1 large carrot, peeled and sliced diagonally
- ✓ ½ cauliflower (around 300g/10½oz), cut into small florets and halved
- ✓ 3 tbsp sunflower or vegetable oil
- ✓ 1 large onion, coarsely grated or very finely chopped
- ✓ 1 tbsp medium or hot curry powder
- ✓ 1 x 227g tin chopped tomatoes
- ✓ 300ml/10fl oz vegetable or chicken stock (made with ½ cube), gluten-free if required
- ✓ 100g/3½oz frozen peas or two large handfuls young spinach leaves, or a mixture
- ✓ plain yoghurt or vegan alternative, to serve
- ✓ mango chutney, to serve

DIRECTIONS:

- ➢ Half-fill a saucepan with cold water and add the potatoes and carrots
- ➢ Bring to the boil and cook for 8 minutes
- ➢ Add the cauliflower florets and cook for 2 minutes more
- ➢ Drain in a colander and set aside.
- ➢ Heat the oil in a large, non-stick frying pan or wide-based saucepan
- ➢ Add the onion and cook over a medium heat for 8 minutes
- ➢ (Or until well softened and lightly browned)
- ➢ Stir regularly. Sprinkle over the curry powder
- ➢ Cook for 30 seconds more, stirring.
- ➢ Add the tomatoes to the onions and cook for 2–3 minutes
- ➢ Stir constantly. Than the stock and bring to a gentle simmer
- ➢ Add the vegetables and peas or spinach and simmer gently for 5 minutes
- ➢ Stir regularly. If the sauce thickens too much, add a splash of water.
- ➢ Serve immediately with yoghurt and mango chutney.

220. HEALTHY CHICKEN TETRAZZINI RECIPE

Servings: 6 **Cook Time: 40 Min** **Prep Time 5 Min**

INGREDIENTS:
- 3 tbsp unsalted butter, divided
- 1 lb chicken tenders
- 8 oz cremini mushrooms, sliced
- 1/2 medium onion, chopped
- 2 large garlic cloves, minced
- 1 1/2 tsp salt, divided
- 1/3 cup all-purpose flour
- 2 cups warm or hot 2% milk
- 1 1/4 cups warm or hot low-sodium chicken stock or broth
- 3/4 cup dry sherry
- 1/4 tsp freshly cracked black pepper
- 1 lb whole-wheat linguine
- 1 1/2 cups shredded 2% milk sharp cheddar cheese

DIRECTIONS:
- Preheat oven to 375 degrees. Grease a 9x9. Bring a large stock pot filled with water to a rolling boil
- Add a generous handful of salt. It should taste as salty as the sea.
- Heat a large skillet with high sides (about two-three inches), to medium heat
- Add one tablespoon of butter
- Season chicken tenders generously with salt and pepepr on both sides
- Once the butter has melted, add the chicken
- Cook until seared on both sides and cooked through, about 2-3 minutes per side
- Remove from the pan, cool and cut into bite-sized pieces.
- Add the remaining two tablespoons butter to the pan
- Then mushrooms, cook without touching for 2-3 minutes until brown
- Stir with a wooden spoon and cook a little bit more
- (Until the other side is brown, about 1-2 minutes)
- Add onion, garlic, and 1/2 teaspoon salt
- Continue to cook until garlic and onion are soft and fragrant, another 2-3 minutes.
- Whisk in flour. Cook for one minute
- Remove from the heat and slowly whisk in warm chicken stock, making sure there are no lumps
- Slowly whisk in milk, dry sherry, and remaining salt along with freshly cracked black pepper
- Return to the heat, bring to a boil and reduce to a simmer
- Simmer until thickened, about 5-7 minutes.
- Once the sauce has simmered for a few minutes and has started to thicken
- Drop the pasta into the boiling water
- Cook until just under aldente. It should have a good bite to it. Drain.
- When the sauce has thickened. Season to taste with salt and pepper
- Add the pasta, 1 cup of the shredded cheese and chopped chicken
- Use tongs to combine everything together. Season to taste again with salt and pepper.
- Transfer to prepared baking dish.
- Cover with remaining 1/2 cup of cheese
- Bake uncovered until hot, bubbly and the cheese has melted, about 20 minutes
- Let sit for 2-3 minutes before serving.

221. SKINNY BRUSCHETTA ZUCCHINI CHIPS

Servings: 6 **Cook Time: 10 Min** **Prep Time 10 Min**

INGREDIENTS:

- ✓ 2 large zucchini, cut into 1/2" slices
- ✓ 1 1/4 cup panko
- ✓ 1 cup Silk unsweetened cashew milk
- ✓ 1/3 cup white whole wheat flour
- ✓ 1/2 teaspoon garlic powder
- ✓ 1/4 teaspoon dry basil
- ✓ 1/3 cup grape seed oil
- ✓ 2 cups cherry tomatoes, finely diced
- ✓ 1/4 cup fresh basil, diced
- ✓ 1 1/2 tablespoons balsamic vinegar
- ✓ 1 1/2 tablespoons olive oil
- ✓ 1 garlic clove, minced
- ✓ Salt to season

DIRECTIONS:

- ➤ Add white whole wheat flour to a large ziplock bag with zucchini slices. Toss to coat.
- ➤ Add Silk Cashew milk to medium bowl, set aside
- ➤ Add panko, dry basil, and garlic powder together. Set aside.
- ➤ Heat large skillet to medium high heat.
- ➤ Add coasted zucchini to milk and then to panko mixture
- ➤ Be sure to coat and press down on both sides so mixture stays on.
- ➤ Add 1/3 cup of grape seed oil to pan, add in coated zucchini chips
- ➤ Saute for 4-5 minutes per side so it is slightly browned
- ➤ Remove and place on paper towel coated plate.
- ➤ Add in the rest of the grape seed oil and the rest of the zucchini chips
- ➤ Cook for the same amount of time
- ➤ Remove and place on plate when finished cooking.
- ➤ In a large bowl add, diced cherry tomatoes, fresh basil
- ➤ Then balsamic vinegar, olive oil, garlic cloves, and salt to taste
- ➤ Toss to mix everything.
- ➤ Serve Zucchini Chips with fresh Bruschetta on top.

222. LIME SORBET SKINNY MARGARITA

Servings: 4 **Cook Time: 0 Min** **Prep Time 10 Min**

INGREDIENTS:

- ✓ 1 lime, cut into 4 slices
- ✓ 1/4 cup sugar
- ✓ 4 cups (2 pints) lime sorbet
- ✓ 4 oz tequila

DIRECTIONS:

- ➤ Start by rubbing the lime wedges around the rims of 4 glasses
- ➤ Place sugar on a small plate and turn each glass upside down
- ➤ Drip the rims in the sugar to coat.
- ➤ Next place 1/2 cup of sorbet in each glass and pour 1 tablespoon of tequila over the top of each glass
- ➤ Serve with a small spoon.

223. *SUPER SKINNY MARGARITA*

Servings: 4 **Cook Time: 0 Min** **Prep Time 10 Min**

INGREDIENTS:

- ✓ 12 ounces Sparkling ICE Lemon Lime water (or any lemon lime flavored sparkling water)
- ✓ 6 ounces tequila
- ✓ 1/4 cup orange juice

- ✓ 2 TBSP fresh squeezed lime juice
- ✓ 1 lime, cut into 4 slices , for garnish
- ✓ Optional: coarse salt for rimming glass

DIRECTIONS:

- ➤ Rub the lime wedges around the rims of 4 glasses
- ➤ Place salt on a small plate
- ➤ Turn each glass upside down, dipping the rims in the sugar to coat
- ➤ Fill glasses with crushed ice.

- ➤ Place sparkling water, tequila, orange juice and lime juice into a pitcher and stir
- ➤ Pour into 4 prepared glasses and garnish with lime slice.

224. *SUNSHINE SKINNY MARGARITA*

Servings: 4 **Cook Time: 0 Min** **Prep Time 10 Min**

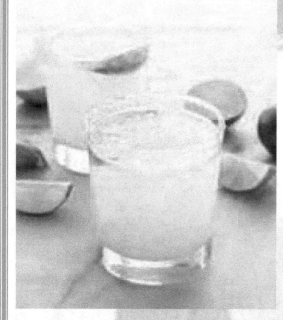

INGREDIENTS:

- ✓ 8 ounces tequila
- ✓ 4 ounces Cointreau
- ✓ 4 ounces fresh orange juice
- ✓ 2 tsp agave (or your choice of sweetener)
- ✓ 1.5 ounces lime juice

SUGGESTED GARNISH

- ✓ 4 slices orange
- ✓ 1.4 cup of sugar for rim of glass

DIRECTIONS:

- ➤ If you are placing sugar on the rim, this step should be done first
- ➤ Wet the edge of the glass with a slice of lime
- ➤ Place the sugar on a small plate
- ➤ Turn each glass upside down and dip the rims in the sugar to coat.
- ➤ Next, fill glasses with ice cubes.
- ➤ Add all ingredients into a pitcher
- ➤ Stir until well combined
- ➤ Poor into glasses and enjoy!

225. LEMON & BUTTERMILK POUND CAKE

Servings: 4 **Cook Time: 55 Min** **Prep Time 10 Min**

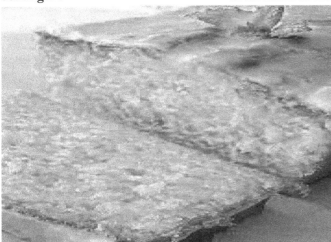

INGREDIENTS:
- ✓ 125g butter, plus extra for the tin
- ✓ 200g plain flour, plus extra for dusting
- ✓ ¼ tsp bicarbonate of soda
- ✓ ¼ tsp baking powder 200g golden caster sugar
- ✓ 4 lemons, finely zested (save a little for the top if you like)
- ✓ 2 large eggs, at room temperature, lightly beaten
- ✓ 100ml buttermilk, at room temperature
- ✓ ½ lemon, juiced For the syrup
- ✓ 50g granulated sugar
- ✓ 2 large lemons, juiced (use the lemons you've zested)

FOR THE ICING
- ✓ 150g icing sugar, sifted 2-3 tbsp lemon juice

DIRECTIONS:
- ➤ Heat oven to 180C/160C fan/gas 4. Butter and flour a loaf tin measuring 22 x 11 x 7cm
- ➤ Sift the flour with a pinch of salt, bicarbonate of soda and baking powder.
- ➤ Beat the butter and sugar until pale and fluffy
- ➤ Then add the lemon zest. Gradually add the eggs a little at a time, beating well after each addition
- ➤ Mix the buttermilk with the lemon juice
- ➤ Fold the flour mixture into the batter, alternating with the buttermilk and lemon mixture.
- ➤ Scrape the batter into the loaf tin and bake for 40-45 mins
- ➤ (Or until a skewer inserted into the centre of the cake comes out clean)
- ➤ Leave to sit for 10 mins, then turn out onto a wire cooling rack with a tray underneath it
- ➤ Set the cake the right way up.
- ➤ To make the syrup, put the ingredients in a small saucepan
- ➤ Heat until the sugar has dissolved
- ➤ Pierce the cake all over with a skewer
- ➤ Then, while the cake is still warm, pour the syrup over slowly. Leave to cool.
- ➤ Gradually add the lemon juice to the icing sugar and mix until just smooth
- ➤ If runny, put in the fridge for about 10 mins
- ➤ Pour or spread the icing over the cake
- ➤ (The bits that drizzle down the side will be caught by the tray under the cooling rack)
- ➤ This icing won't set hard, but do leave it to set a little before serving.

226. GINGER & WHITE CHOCOLATE CAKE

Servings: 4   **Cook Time: 55 Min**   **Prep Time 10 Min**

INGREDIENTS:

- ✓ 220g unsalted butter , softened 365g self-raising flour
- ✓ 200g muscovado sugar 50g black treacle
- ✓ 150g golden syrup
- ✓ 2 large eggs , lightly beaten 300ml milk
- ✓ 2 balls stem ginger in syrup, finely chopped, plus 50ml of the syrup
- ✓ 1 tsp fine sea salt
- ✓ 3 tsp ground ginger
- ✓ ½ tsp cinnamon
- ✓ ½ tsp bicarbonate of soda
- ✓ small handful of crystallised ginger pieces, chopped, to decorate For the white chocolate icing
- ✓ 30ml milk
- ✓ 160g icing sugar , sieved
- ✓ 150g white chocolate , chopped

DIRECTIONS:

- ➢ Heat the oven to 180C/160C fan/gas 4. Melt 1 tbsp butter in a small pan
- ➢ Then stir in ½ tbsp flour to create a wet paste
- ➢ Brush it over the inside of a 9-inch bundt tin
- ➢ Put the remaining butter, sugar, treacle and golden syrup in a pan set over a medium heat
- ➢ Stir until everything has melted together. Leave to cool a little.
- ➢ Pour the mixture into a large bowl
- ➢ Whisk in the eggs and milk. Fold in the stem ginger, remaining flour, salt, ground ginger, cinnamon and bicarb

- ➢ Tip into the prepared tin and bake for 40-45 mins
- ➢ (Or until firm to the touch)
- ➢ Leave to cool for 10 mins in the tin
- ➢ Then turn out onto a wire rack to cool completely.
- ➢ To make the icing, whisk the milk, ginger syrup and icing sugar together. Melt the chocolate in a heatproof bowl in the microwave in 1-min bursts. Leave to cool a little, then whisk into the milk mixture
- ➢ Spoon the icing over the cake
- ➢ Then decorate with the crystallised ginger pieces.

227. PEANUT BUTTER & JAM FLAPJACKS

Servings: 4   **Cook Time: 30 Min**   **Prep Time 10 Min**

INGREDIENTS:

- ✓ 5 tbsp salted butter , plus extra for the tin
- ✓ 250g crunchy peanut butter
- ✓ 8 tbsp strawberry or raspberry jam

- ✓ 80g light brown soft sugar
- ✓ 200g rolled oats

DIRECTIONS:

- ➢ Heat the oven to 180C/160C fan/gas 4
- ➢ Butter and line the base and sides of a 20cm square cake tin with baking parchment.
- ➢ Put 3 tbsp each of the peanut butter and jam in separate small bowls and set aside
- ➢ Tip the remaining peanut butter, the rest of the jam and the butter
- ➢ Than sugar into a pan set over a medium heat
- ➢ Stir until everything has melted together.

- ➢ Quickly stir in the oats, then leave to cool for 5 mins.
- ➢ Spoon the mixture into the prepared cake tin
- ➢ Gently press down with your hands
- ➢ Dot over the reserved peanut butter and jam
- ➢ Then bake for 20-25 mins or until golden brown
- ➢ Leave to cool completely in the tin
- ➢ Then turn out onto a board and cut into squares.

228. INSTANT FROZEN BERRY YOGURT

Servings: 4   **Cook Time: 0 Min**   **Prep Time 30 Min**

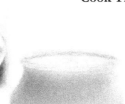

INGREDIENTS:

- ✓ 250g frozen mixed berry
- ✓ 250g 0%-fat Greek yogurt
- ✓ 1 tbsp honey or agave syrup

DIRECTIONS:

- ➢ Blend berries, yogurt and honey or agave syrup in a food processor for 20 seconds
- ➢ (Until it comes together to a smooth ice-cream texture)
- ➢ Scoop into bowls and serve.

229. QUICK PRAWN, COCONUT & TOMATO CURRY

Servings: 4   **Cook Time: 0 Min**   **Prep Time 30 Min**

INGREDIENTS:

- ✓ 2 tbsp vegetable oil
- ✓ 1 medium onion , thinly sliced
- ✓ 2 garlic cloves , sliced
- ✓ 1 green chilli , deseeded and sliced
- ✓ 3 tbsp curry paste
- ✓ 1 tbsp tomato purée
- ✓ 200ml vegetable stock
- ✓ 200ml coconut cream
- ✓ 350g raw prawn
- ✓ Coriander sprigs and rice, to serve

DIRECTIONS:

- ➢ Heat the oil in a large frying pan
- ➢ Fry the onion, garlic and half the chilli for 5 mins or until softened
- ➢ Add the curry paste and cook for 1 min more
- ➢ Then the tomato purée, stock and coconut cream.
- ➢ Simmer on medium heat for 10 mins add the prawns.
- ➢ Cook for 3 mins or until they turn opaque
- ➢ Scatter on the remaining green chillies and coriander sprigs
- ➢ Then serve with rice

230. PARMESAN CRUSTED SALMON

Serving: 1 **Cook Time: 15Min** **Prep Time 10 Min**

INGREDIENTS

- ✓ Broccoli crowns
- ✓ Olive oil
- ✓ Garlic
- ✓ Salt and pepper
- ✓ Skinless salmon fillets
- ✓ Mayonnaise
- ✓ Lemon juice
- ✓ Grated Parmesan
- ✓ Bread crumbs
- ✓ Fresh parsley
- ✓ Lemon zest
- ✓ Dried thyme

DIRECTIONS

- ➢ Place broccoli on a foil-lined baking sheet in a mound.
- ➢ Drizzle with olive oil and season with salt and pepper
- ➢ Then toss to coat. Spread broccoli to edges of baking sheet.
- ➢ Season salmon with salt and pepper
- ➢ Place in center of baking tray
- ➢ Whisk together mayo, lemon juice and garlic and brush over salmon.
- ➢ In a separate bowl, whisk together bread crumbs
- ➢ Add Parmesan, parsley, lemon zest, thyme and olive oil
- ➢ Sprinkle over salmon.
- ➢ Bake until salmon is cooked and broccoli is crisp-tender

Note: Unsure what the correct salmon bake time is? This recipe calls for you to bake salmon in a 400-degree F oven for 12 to 15 minutes. You'll know the salmon is done baking when it's easy to flake with a fork.

231. SLOW-COOKER CHEESY ITALIAN TORTELLINI

Servings: 4 **Cook Time: 4 H 30Min** **Prep Time 15 Min**

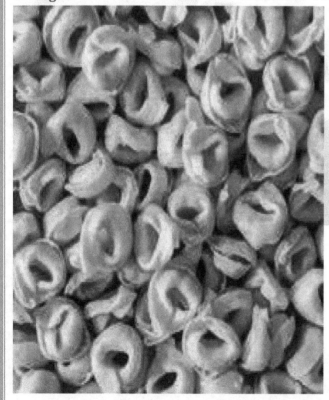

INGREDIENTS

- ✓ ½ lb lean (at least 80%) ground beef
- ✓ ½ lb bulk Italian sausage
- ✓ 1 container (15 oz) refrigerated marinara sauce
- ✓ 1 cup sliced fresh mushrooms
- ✓ 1 can (14.5 oz) diced tomatoes with Italian herbs, undrained
- ✓ 1 package (9 oz) refrigerated cheese-filled tortellini
- ✓ 1 cup shredded mozzarella cheese or pizza cheese blend (4 oz)

DIRECTIONS

- ➢ Prevent your screen from going dark while you cook.
- ➢ In 10-inch skillet, cook beef and sausage over medium-high heat 5 to 7 minutes
- ➢ Stirring occasionally, until brown; drain.
- ➢ Spray inside of 4- to 5 quart slow cooker with cooking spray
- ➢ Mix beef mixture, marinara sauce, mushrooms and tomatoes in cooker
- ➢ Cover; cook on Low heat setting 7 to 8 hours.
- ➢ Stir in tortellini; sprinkle with cheese
- ➢ Cover; cook on Low heat setting about 15 minutes longer
- ➢ (Or until tortellini are tender)

232. ONE-PAN ITALIAN SAUSAGE AND PEPPERS PASTA

Servings: 4   **Cook Time: 4 H 30Min**   **Prep Time 15 Min**

INGREDIENTS

- 2 Tablespoons extra virgin olive oil
- 4 raw Italian sausage links, cut in half
- 1 green bell pepper, sliced
- 1 large shallot or 1/2 small onion, chopped
- 2 cloves garlic, minced
- Salt and pepper
- 2 cups chicken broth

- 1-1/4 cups really good marinara sauce (locals use Gino's)
- 1/2 teaspoon Italian Seasoning
- 1/4 teaspoon red chili pepper flakes (optional)
- 1/2lb penne pasta (gluten-free if you need it)
- 4 thin slices provolone cheese

DIRECTIONS

- Heat oil in a large, nonstick pan over medium-high heat
- Add sausages then brown on both sides
- (They do not need to be cooked all the way through)
- Remove to a plate then set aside.
- Turn heat down to medium
- Then add peppers and shallots to pan
- Season with salt and pepper then saute for 5 minutes
- (Or until peppers are crisp-tender)
- Add garlic then saute for 30 more seconds.
- Join also chicken broth, marinara sauce Italian seasoning, red chili pepper flakes to pan
- Then turn heat up to bring mixture to a boil

- Add pasta then shake pan to cover all the pasta with liquid and then nestle sausages on top
- Place a lid on top then reduce heat to medium-low and simmer for 8-10 minutes
- (Or until pasta is just under al dente)
- Shake the pan every so often to make sure the pasta is cooking evenly
- Don't let the pasta reach al dente as it still has a few more minutes to cook.
- Arrange cheese slices on top of pasta and sausages
- Then place lid back on top.
- Let cheese melt then remove pan from heat Let sit with the lid off to thicken slightly for a few minutes before serving.

Servings: 4 **Cook Time: 20 Min** **Prep Time 15 Min**

INGREDIENTS

- ✓ 4 x 125g/4oz salmon fillets, with skin left on
- ✓ 2 heaped tbsp hoisin sauce (from a jar or bottle)
- ✓ 150g/5½oz cherry tomatoes, halved
- ✓ 140g/5oz medium egg noodles
- ✓ 200g/7oz long-stemmed broccoli, trimmed
- ✓ Freshly ground black pepper
- ✓ Dark soy sauce, to serve (optional)

DIRECTIONS

- ➢ Preheat the oven to 220C/200C Fan/Gas 7 and line a small, shallow ovenproof dish with kitchen foil.
- ➢ Place the salmon fillets into the dish, skin-side down
- ➢ Brush generously with the hoisin sauce
- ➢ Make sure the fillets are placed at least 5cm/2in apart from each other
- ➢ Scatter the cherry tomatoes around them.
- ➢ Cook for 15 minutes, or until the salmon is cooked through.
- ➢ Meanwhile, prepare the noodles

- ➢ Half-fill a saucepan with water and bring to the boil
- ➢ Add the noodles, return to the boil and cook for 1 minute
- ➢ Stir to separate the strands
- ➢ Add the broccoli and cook for 3 more minutes, stirring occasionally.
- ➢ Divide the noodles and broccoli between four warmed plates
- ➢ Top with the salmon fillets and scatter with the cherry tomatoes
- ➢ Season with pepper and serve sprinkled with a little soy sauce, if using

Servings: 5   **Cook Time: 30 Min**   **Prep Time 15 Min**

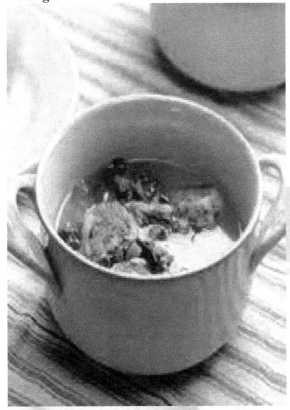

INGREDIENTS

FOR THE MEATBALLS

- ✓ 1/2 lb. chicken hearts
- ✓ 1/4 c. cooked soybeans
- ✓ 1 clove garlic, grated
- ✓ 2 shishito peppers, diced
- ✓ 1/4 c. parsley leaves
- ✓ 1/4 c. walnuts
- ✓ 1 tsp. gochugaru
- ✓ 1/2 tsp. mushroom powder
- ✓ 1/4 tsp. kosher salt

FOR THE SOUP

- ✓ 2 tbsp. extra-virgin olive oil
- ✓ 2 c. diced cauliflower stems or bite-sized florets
- ✓ 1 c. packed chopped kale
- ✓ 1/2 c. soybeans
- ✓ 8 shishito peppers, sliced
- ✓ 1 tsp. steak seasoning
- ✓ 1/4 tsp. freshly ground black pepper
- ✓ 1/4 tsp. ground white pepper
- ✓ 5 c. homemade bone broth or low-sodium chicken broth
- ✓ 1 tsp. citrus herb seasoning blend
- ✓ 1/8 tsp. MSG (optional)
- ✓ Freshly chopped parsley, for serving

DIRECTIONS

➢ Make the meatballs: In a food processor, combine all ingredients and pulse until a mostly smooth paste forms
➢ Transfer to a large bowl and let chill in the refrigerator.
➢ Make the soup: In a large pot over medium heat, heat oil
➢ dd cauliflower, kale, soybeans, and peppers and cook
➢ (Stirring occasionally, until cauliflower is knife-tender)
➢ Add steak seasoning, pepper, white pepper, and stir to evenly distribute

➢ Then broth, herb seasoning, and MSG (if using) to a simmer
➢ Let cook 10 minutes to reduce slightly.
➢ Using two small spoons, scoop out meatballs and drop them directly into the simmering broth
➢ Let simmer until meatballs are fully cooked, about 10 minutes.
➢ Garnish with parsley before serving.
➢ If the spoons become too sticky with the meatball mixture, dip them into a small bowl of cold water for an easier release.

235. STUFFED SPLEEN

Servings: 2   **Cook Time: 45 Min**   **Prep Time 15 Min**

INGREDIENTS
- ✓ 2 pork spleens, fat trimmed and reserved
- ✓ 4 cloves garlic, sliced
- ✓ 3 c. packed finely chopped kale (about 1/2 bunch)
- ✓ 1 tsp. steak seasoning
- ✓ 1/2 c. cooked soybeans, roughly chopped
- ✓ Extra-virgin olive oil
- ✓ 12 shishito peppers Kosher salt
- ✓ Freshly chopped parsley, for garnish

DIRECTIONS
- ➢ Cook the kale: In a cast iron skillet over medium heat, render spleen fat, about 3 minutes.
- ➢ Transfer crispy spleen bits to a bowl, then add garlic to skillet
- ➢ Stir and cook until lightly golden
- ➢ Then add kale and steak seasoning and cook until wilted, about 5 minutes. Add soybeans and cook for 5 minutes more
- ➢ Transfer mixture to a bowl and let cool.
- ➢ On a cutting board, use a sharp paring knife to create a long pocket inside each spleen by partially butterflying the spleen
- ➢ Stuff each spleen with kale mixture
- ➢ Then use toothpicks to pin the spleen shut.
- ➢ Preheat oven to 375°. In a cast iron skillet over medium heat, heat 2 teaspoons oil
- ➢ Add spleens and let sear 5 minutes per side
- ➢ Then transfer skillet to the oven and bake until internal temperature reaches 160°, about 10 minutes
- ➢ Transfer to a cutting board and let rest 10 minutes before slicing.
- ➢ Meanwhile, return skillet to medium heat and heat 1 teaspoon oil
- ➢ Add shishitos and let cook until peppers are lightly blistered
- ➢ Season with salt.
- ➢ Serve sliced spleen with blistered shishitos
- ➢ Garnish with parsley before serving if desired.

236. SKINNY GINGERBREAD MEN

Servings: 6   **Cook Time: 25 Min**   **Prep Time 15 Min**

INGREDIENTS
- ✓ 1/4 cup butter, softened
- ✓ 1/2 cup packed brown sugar
- ✓ 3/4 cup dark molasses
- ✓ 1/3 cup cold water
- ✓ 3 1/2 cups all-purpose flour, or half all-purpose, half whole wheat
- ✓ 1 tsp. baking soda
- ✓ 2 tsp. cinnamon
- ✓ 1 tsp. ground ginger
- ✓ 1/2 tsp. allspice
- ✓ 1/2 tsp. salt
- ✓ 1/4 tsp. ground cloves

DIRECTIONS
- ➢ In a large bowl, beat butter, brown sugar, molasses and water with an electric mixer or by hand until smooth
- ➢ In another large bowl, stir together the flour, baking soda, cinnamon, ginger, allspice, salt and cloves.
- ➢ Add the flour mixture to the molasses mixture
- ➢ Stir by hand just until you have a soft dough
- ➢ Divide the dough in half, shape each piece into a disc, wrap in plastic
- ➢ Refrigerate for 2 hours or up to a few days.
- ➢ When you're ready to bake, preheat the oven to 350°F.
- ➢ On a lightly floured surface or between two pieces of waxed or parchment paper, roll one piece of dough out about 1/8" thick
- ➢ Cut out with cookie cutters
- ➢ Place about an inch apart on a cookie sheet that has been sprayed with nonstick spray.
- ➢ Bake for 12–15 minutes, until set.
- ➢ Bake a few minutes longer for crispier cookies
- ➢ Transfer to a wire rack to cool
- ➢ Repeat with remaining dough, rerolling scraps once to get as many cookies as possible
- ➢ Makes 3 dozen cookies.

237. CHICKEN HEART KALE BREAKFAST CUPS

Servings: 6   Cook Time: 30 Min   Prep Time 15 Min

INGREDIENTS

FOR THE MASSAGED KALE
- ✓ 4 c. packed kale leaves
- ✓ 1 tbsp. extra-virgin olive oil

FOR THE CHICKEN HEARTS
- ✓ 2 tbsp. extra-virgin olive oil
- ✓ 4 cloves garlic, sliced
- ✓ 4 shishito peppers, finely chopped
- ✓ 8 oz. chicken hearts, quartered Kosher salt

FOR SERVING
- ✓ Soft scrambled eggs Crumbled feta

- ✓ 1 tsp. mixed herb seasoning blend Kosher salt
- ✓ Freshly ground black pepper

- ✓ 1 tsp. cumin seeds
- ✓ Freshly ground black pepper
- ✓ 1/4 tsp. ground white pepper (optional)
- ✓ 1 tsp. togarashi (optional)

- ✓ Everything bagel seasoning (optional)

DIRECTIONS

- ➢ Make the massaged kale: In a large bowl, using your hands, toss to combine all ingredients
- ➢ Rub with your fingers to massage oil
- ➢ Season into kale. Season with more salt and pepper if desired, then set aside.
- ➢ Make the chicken hearts: In a large skillet over medium heat, heat oil
- ➢ Add garlic and peppers and stir until fragrant and softened
- ➢ Then add chicken hearts. Cook until hearts begin to turn golden and develop crispy edges

- ➢ Then add in cumin, pepper, white pepper, and togarashi, if using
- ➢ Stir until spices are toasted, about 1 minute.
- ➢ Assemble cups: Top each piece of kale with scrambled eggs, chicken hearts, feta, and everything bagel seasoning, if using.
- ➢ For a cleaner flavor, blanch your chicken hearts in boiling water briefly, about 1 minute
- ➢ Then drain and rinse and let cool before proceeding with the recipe.

238. SKINNY TACO DIP

Servings: 24   Cook Time: 0 Min   Prep Time 20 Min

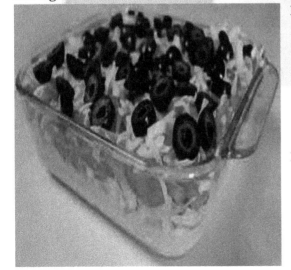

INGREDIENTS
- ✓ 8 oz 1/3 less fat Philadelphia cream cheese
- ✓ 8 oz reduced fat sour cream
- ✓ 16 oz jar mild salsa
- ✓ 1/2 packet taco seasoning, check for GF
- ✓ 2 cups iceberg lettuce, shredded fine
- ✓ 2 large tomatoes, seeds removed and diced
- ✓ 1 cup reduced fat shredded cheddar cheese
- ✓ 2.25 oz sliced black olives

DIRECTIONS
- ➢ In a large bowl combine cream cheese, sour cream, salsa and taco seasoning
- ➢ Mix well with an electric mixer.
- ➢ Spread on the bottom of a large shallow glass dish.
- ➢ Top with shredded lettuce, tomatoes, shredded cheese and black olives
- ➢ Serve with baked tortilla chips

Servings: 2   **Cook Time: 30 Min**   **Prep Time 15 Min**

INGREDIENTS

FOR THE GARLIC CHIPS
- ✓ 1 tbsp. extra-virgin olive oil
- ✓ 1 head garlic, peeled and thinly sliced Kosher salt

FOR THE TOASTY SOYBEANS
- ✓ 1/2 c. soaked soybeans, patted dry
- ✓ 6 shishito peppers, thinly sliced
- ✓ 1 tbsp. low-sodium soy sauce

FOR THE EGG NOODLES
- ✓ 6 large eggs
- ✓ 2 large egg yolks
- ✓ 1/8 tsp. kosher salt
- ✓ 1 tsp. togarashi (optional)
- ✓ Extra-virgin olive oil, for pan

FOR THE BROTH
- ✓ 4 c. homemade bone broth or low-sodium chicken or vegetable broth
- ✓ 3 cloves grated garlic
- ✓ Kosher salt
- ✓ Freshly ground black pepper
- ✓ 1/4 tsp. ground white pepper
- ✓ 1/8 tsp. MSG (optional)

DIRECTIONS

- ➢ Make the garlic chips: In a medium skillet over medium heat, heat oil
- ➢ Add garlic and spread into a single layer with minimal overlapping
- ➢ Let cook until garlic begins to turn lightly golden
- ➢ Then begin to stir frequently to ensure even heating
- ➢ Remove from heat when most garlic pieces are nicely golden
- ➢ Transfer the garlic to a plate and keeping the oil in the skillet.
- ➢ Make toasty soybeans: Return skillet with oil to medium heat
- ➢ Add in soybeans and peppers and stir-fry
- ➢ (Until soybeans are toasty and peppers are slightly charred)
- ➢ Add in soy sauce and stir to combine until warmed through
- ➢ Remove from heat.
- ➢ Make the egg noodles: In a medium bowl
- ➢ Whisk together eggs and yolks with salt and togarashi, if using
- ➢ In a cast-iron or nonstick pan over medium- low heat, heat 1 teaspoon oil
- ➢ Use a small piece of paper towel to evenly coat the bottom of the pan with oil
- ➢ Pour in just enough egg mixture to form a thin layer on the bottom of the pan
- ➢ Twirl the pan to ensure even coverage as the egg sets
- ➢ Let cook until bottom is lightly golden, about 1 minute
- ➢ Then use an offset spatula to release the edge of the egg from the pan
- ➢ Use your hands or a rubber spatula to help, gently flip the egg
- ➢ Let the second side cook until set, about 30 seconds to 1 minute
- ➢ Transfer cooked egg to a plate and repeat process with remaining egg mixture.
- ➢ Stack your sheets of cooked egg together on a cutting board
- ➢ Then roll into a log. Using a sharp chef's knife, cut into noodles.
- ➢ Meanwhile, make broth: In a large pot over medium heat
- ➢ Add all broth ingredients and bring to a boil. Let simmer for about 5 minutes.
- ➢ Place egg noodles into serving bowls, then ladle broth over
- ➢ Top with toasty soybeans and garlic chips before serving.
- ➢ To make it a heartier meal, you can top your bowl of noodles with any leftovers or additional toppings!

Servings: 20   **Cook Time: 45 Min**   **Prep Time 10 Min**

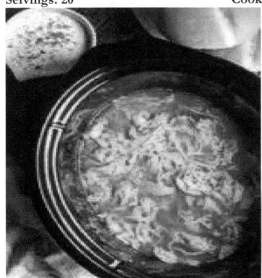

INGREDIENTS

INGREDIENTS FOR FALAFEL

- ✓ 1/2 medium yellow onion, cut into quarters
- ✓ 4 cloves garlic
- ✓ 1/4 c. packed parsley leaves
- ✓ 1/4 c. packed cilantro leaves
- ✓ 2 (15-oz.) cans chickpeas, rinsed and drained
- ✓ 1 tsp. kosher salt
- ✓ 1 tsp. baking powder
- ✓ 1 tsp. dried coriander
- ✓ 1/2 tsp. crushed red pepper flakes

FOR TAHINI SAUCE

- ✓ 1/3 c. tahini
- ✓ Juice of 1/2 a lemon
- ✓ 3 tbsp. water, plus more as needed Pinch kosher salt
- ✓ Pinch red pepper flakes

DIRECTIONS

- ➢ In a food processor, pulse onion, garlic, parsley, and cilantro
- ➢ (Until roughly chopped)
- ➢ Scrap down sides as needed
- ➢ Add drained chickpeas, salt, baking powder, coriander, cumin, and red pepper flakes
- ➢ Pulse again until chickpeas are mostly broken down with some chunks
- ➢ You can stop just before the mixture turns into a paste
- ➢ Taste and adjust seasonings.
- ➢ Scoop out about 2 tablespoons worth of mixture
- ➢ Gently form into a ball without squeezing together too much or falafels will be dense

- ➢ Working in batches, place falafels in basket of air fryer
- ➢ Cook at 370° for 15 minutes.
- ➢ Meanwhile, make tahini sauce: In a medium bowl, combine tahini and lemon juice
- ➢ Add water and stir until combined
- ➢ Then more water 1 tablespoon at a time until desired consistency is reached
- ➢ Season with a big pinch of salt and red pepper flakes.
- ➢ Serve falafels as is with sauce, in a salad, or in a pita.

241. VEGAN TACO SALAD

Servings: 6   **Cook Time: 30 Min**   **Prep Time 10 Min**

INGREDIENTS

FOR SALAD

- ✓ 2 c. water
- ✓ 1 c. quinoa
- ✓ 1 (15-oz.) can black beans, rinsed and drained
- ✓ 1 (15-oz.) can pinto beans, rinsed and drained
- ✓ 1 c. corn

FOR AVOCADO-CHIPOTLE DRESSING

- ✓ 2 large avocados, pitted
- ✓ 1 chipotle in adobo sauce, plus 1 tsp. sauce Juice of 1 lime
- ✓ 1/4 c. fresh cilantro
- ✓ 2 cloves garlic

- ✓ 1 tbsp. taco seasoning Kosher salt
- ✓ Freshly ground black pepper Chopped romaine
- ✓ 1/2 small red onion, thinly sliced
- ✓ 1 c. cherry tomatoes, halved
- ✓ 1bell pepper, chopped Tortilla chips

- ✓ 1/4 c. water
- ✓ 2 tbsp. extra-virgin olive oil
- ✓ 2 tbsp. white wine vinegar Kosher salt
- ✓ Freshly ground black pepper

DIRECTIONS

- ➤ In a medium pot over medium heat, bring water to a boil
- ➤ Add Quinoa, reduce heat to a simmer, then cover and cook 12 minutes
- ➤ (Or until water is absorbed)
- ➤ Remove from heat, but keep covered for 5 minutes.
- ➤ Add beans, corn, and taco seasoning to warm Quinoa
- ➤ Toss to combine. Season with salt and pepper.

- ➤ In a blender or small food processor, blend together dressing ingredients
- ➤ Season with salt and pepper
- ➤ Add more vinegar or water to thin dressing as desired.
- ➤ In a large bowl, add romaine and toss with quinoa mixture
- ➤ Then red onions, tomatoes, and bell pepper
- ➤ Serve with chipotle dressing and tortilla chips.

242. ONE POT MUSHROOM SPINACH ARTICHOKE PASTA

Servings: 6   **Cook Time: 20 Min**   **Prep Time 5 Min**

INGREDIENTS

- ✓ 12 ounces fettuccine
- ✓ 1 (14-ounce) can quartered artichoke hearts, drained
- ✓ 8 ounces cremini mushrooms, thinly sliced
- ✓ 1 large onion, thinly sliced 2 cloves garlic, thinly sliced
- ✓ 1/2 teaspoon dried basil

- ✓ 1/4 teaspoon dried thyme
- ✓ 1/4 teaspoon crushed red pepper flakes, optional
- ✓ Kosher salt and freshly ground black pepper, to taste
- ✓ 2 cups baby spinach
- ✓ 1 cup freshly grated Parmesan
- ✓ 2 tablespoons unsalted butter

DIRECTIONS

- ➤ In a large stockpot or Dutch oven over medium high heat
- ➤ Combine fettuccine, artichoke hearts, mushrooms, onion, garlic, basil, thyme
- ➤ Then red pepper flakes and 4 1/2 cups water
- ➤ Season with salt and pepper, to taste.

- ➤ Bring to a boil; reduce heat and simmer, uncovered
- ➤ (Until pasta is cooked through and liquid has reduced, about 12-15 minutes)
- ➤ Stir in spinach, Parmesan and butter
- ➤ (Until the spinach has wilted, about 2-3 minutes)
- ➤ Serve immediately.

243. PULLED PORK SANDWICHES WITH APPLE SLAW

Servings: 6 **Cook Time: 12 H** **Prep Time 5 Min**

INGREDIENTS
FOR PULLED PORK
- ✓ 3 lb boneless pork shoulder 2 tsp paprika
- ✓ 1 tsp cumin
- ✓ 1 tsp garlic powder
- ✓ 1/8 tsp cayenne pepper optional 2 tsp salt
- ✓ 1 tsp ground black pepper
- ✓ 1/2 cup apple cider vinegar
- ✓ 1/4 cup honey 2 tbsp olive oil
- ✓ 2 tbsp tomato paste
- ✓ 1 tsp Worcestershire sauce
- ✓ 1 onion roughly sliced
- ✓ 8 rolls or buns for serving

FOR APPLE SLAW
- ✓ 2 apples julienned
- ✓ 2 cups cabbage shredded
- ✓ 2 carrots julienned
- ✓ 3 green onions chopped
- ✓ 2 tbsp Greek yogurt
- ✓ 3 tbsp apple cider vinegar
- ✓ 2 tsp honey
- ✓ 2 tsp dijon mustard
- ✓ 3 tbsp poppy seeds
- ✓ 1/2 lemon juiced
- ✓ 1 clove garlic
- ✓ Salt and Pepper to taste

DIRECTIONS
- ➢ In a small bowl, stir the paprika, cumin, garlic powder, cayenne pepper
- ➢ Add salt, pepper, apple cider vinegar, honey, olive oil, tomato paste
- ➢ Worcestershire sauce until well combined.
- ➢ Place the onions at the bottom of a slow cooker
- ➢ Add the pork on top and pour the sauce over it
- ➢ Make sure to cover the entire piece of meat
- ➢ Some of the sauce may drip to the bottom of the slow cooker.
- ➢ Turn the slow cooker on and cook for 4 hours on high or 8 hours on low.
- ➢ In the meantime, make the apple slaw by stirring together in a small bowl the Greek yogurt, apple cider vinegar
- ➢ Add honey, dijon mustard, poppy seeds, lemon juice, garlic, salt and pepper together.
- ➢ In a large bowl toss the apples, cabbage, carrots and green onions together
- ➢ Add the slaw dressing and toss until completed coated
- ➢ Place in fridge and let chill until ready to serve
- ➢ This slaw will keep for a couple of days and is perfect for leftovers.
- ➢ When pork is cooked all the way through, take it out of the slow cooker and let cool slightly
- ➢ Shred pork into small pieces using 2 forks. Discard onions.
- ➢ Add some or all of the sauce back into the shredded pork
- ➢ To serve, cut buns in half, spoon a huge serving of pork onto the bottom bun
- ➢ Top with a spoonful of the apple slaw and top with the remaining piece of bun

Notes: Yield: Roughly 12 slider size or 8 regular sandwiches Storage: store pork in air-tight container in fridge for a week, for slaw store in air-tight container for up to 3 days.

244. ONE POT CREAMY SAUSAGE GNOCCHI

Servings: 6   **Cook Time: 20 Min**   **Prep Time 10 Min**

INGREDIENTS

- ✓ 1 lb mild ground sausage
- ✓ 1 onion diced
- ✓ 2 cloves garlic minced
- ✓ 1 tsp salt
- ✓ 1 tsp pepper
- ✓ 2 tsp Italian seasoning
- ✓ 1 tsp garlic powder

- ✓ 1 15 oz can garlic and olive oil petite diced tomatoes (any flavor will do)
- ✓ 3/4 cup heavy cream
- ✓ 1 16 oz pkg gnocchi
- ✓ 2-3 cups spinach
- ✓ 1 1-2 cup shredded mozzarella cheese
- ✓ Parsley for garnish optional

DIRECTIONS

- ➢ In skillet over medium high heat add your sausage, onion, garlic
- ➢ Season and saute until browned
- ➢ Add in your tomatoes, creamy, gnocchi, spinach

- ➢ Heat until gnocchi is cooked, spinach is wilted and some of the cream has reduced (about 8-10 minutes)
- ➢ Stir in your shredded mozzarella cheese until melted
- ➢ Top with more cheese and parsley if desired.

245. EASY CHICKEN TORTELLINI SOUP

Servings: 6   **Cook Time: 25 Min**   **Prep Time 10 Min**

INGREDIENTS

- ✓ Chopped parsley to taste1 tablespoon olive oil
- ✓ 1/2 medium onion chopped
- ✓ 3 sticks celery finely chopped
- ✓ 3 large carrots peeled & sliced or chopped
- ✓ 2 cloves garlic minced
- ✓ 8 cups chicken broth
- ✓ 2 dashes Italian seasoning
- ✓ 2 cups cooked chicken (or more, to taste)
- ✓ 1 (20 ounce) package refrigerated cheese tortellini
- ✓ Salt & pepper to taste

DIRECTIONS

- ➢ Chop your onion. Add it to a large soup pot along with the olive oil
- ➢ Sauté over medium-high heat for 5-7 minutes (ok if onion lightly browns).
- ➢ Meanwhile, chop the celery and carrots
- ➢ Then add them to the pot along with the garlic
- ➢ Give it a good stir and cook for a couple minutes.
- ➢ Add the chicken broth and Italian seasoning
- ➢ Increase the heat to high, and once it starts to boil, reduce the heat to a rapid simmer and let it cook for 10 minutes.

- ➢ Add the chicken and tortellini to the pot
- ➢ Increase the heat to medium-high and let the soup cook for another 10 minutes or so
- ➢ If it starts to boil furiously, you may need to turn the heat down again.
- ➢ Season with salt & pepper as needed
- ➢ Garnish with the chopped parsley. Serve immediately.

NOTES: Time for cooking chicken: Use 3-4 raw chicken breasts or 6 chicken thighs and cook it on low for 6-8 hours or high for 3-4 hours (test to make sure the chicken is cooked through and shreds easily). Then, add the tortellini in with about 30 minutes to go.

246. AIR FRYER FALAFEL

Servings: 20　　　　**Cook Time: 35 Min**　　　　**Prep Time 10 Min**

INGREDIENTS
FOR FALAFEL
- ✓ 1/2 medium yellow onion, cut into quarters
- ✓ 4 cloves garlic
- ✓ 1/4 c. packed parsley leaves
- ✓ 1/4 c. packed cilantro leaves
- ✓ 2 (15-oz.) cans chickpeas, rinsed and drained

FOR TAHINI SAUCE
- ✓ 1/3 c. tahini
- ✓ Juice of 1/2 a lemon
- ✓ 3 tbsp. water, plus more as needed

- ✓ 1 tsp. kosher salt
- ✓ 1 tsp. baking powder
- ✓ 1 tsp. dried coriander
- ✓ 1/2 tsp. crushed red pepper flakes

- ✓ Pinch kosher salt
- ✓ Pinch red pepper flakes

DIRECTIONS
- ➢ In a food processor, pulse onion, garlic, parsley, and cilantro
- ➢ (Until roughly chopped, scraping down sides as needed)
- ➢ Add drained chickpeas, salt, baking powder, coriander, cumin, and red pepper flakes
- ➢ Pulse again until chickpeas are mostly broken down with some chunks
- ➢ You can stop just before the mixture turns into a paste
- ➢ Taste and adjust seasonings.
- ➢ Scoop out about 2 tablespoons worth of mixture

- ➢ Gently form into a ball without squeezing together too much or falafels will be dense
- ➢ Working in batches, place falafels in basket of air fryer and cook at 370° for 15 minutes.
- ➢ Meanwhile, make tahini sauce: In a medium bowl, combine tahini and lemon juice
- ➢ Add water and stir until combined.
- ➢ Then more water 1 tablespoon at a time until desired consistency is reached. Season with a big pinch of salt and red pepper flakes.
- ➢ Serve falafels as is with sauce, in a salad, or in a pita

247. AIR FRYER CHICKEN PARMESAN

Servings: 4　　　　**Cook Time: 40 Min**　　　　**Prep Time 10 Min**

INGREDIENTS
- ✓ 2 large boneless chicken breasts
- ✓ Kosher salt
- ✓ Freshly ground black pepper
- ✓ 1/3 c. all-purpose flour
- ✓ 2 large eggs
- ✓ 1 c. panko bread crumbs
- ✓ 1/4 c. freshly grated Parmesan

- ✓ 1 tsp. dried oregano
- ✓ 1/2 tsp. garlic powder
- ✓ 1/2 tsp. crushed red pepper flakes
- ✓ 1 c. marinara sauce
- ✓ 1 c. shredded mozzarella
- ✓ Freshly chopped parsley, for garnish

DIRECTIONS
- ➢ Carefully butterfly chicken by cutting in half widthwise to create 4 thin pieces of chicken
- ➢ Season on both sides with salt and pepper.
- ➢ Prepare dredging station: Place flour in a shallow bowl
- ➢ Season with a large pinch of salt and pepper
- ➢ Place eggs in a second bowl and beat
- ➢ In a third bowl, combine bread crumbs, Parmesan, oregano, garlic powder, and red pepper flakes.
- ➢ Working with one piece of a chicken at a time, coat in flour

- ➢ Then dip in eggs, and finally press into panko mixture
- ➢ Make sure both sides are coated well.
- ➢ Working in batches as necessary
- ➢ Place chicken in basket of air fryer
- ➢ Cook at 400° for 5 minutes on each side
- ➢ Top chicken with sauce and mozzarella
- ➢ Cook at 400° for 3 minutes more
- ➢ (Or until cheese is melty and golden)
- ➢ Garnish with parsley to serve.

248. SHEET PAN PARMESAN, PARMESAN CHICKEN AND BROCCOLI

Servings: 4 **Cook Time: 20 Min** **Prep Time 15 Min**

INGREDIENTS

- ✓ 2 cups broccoli florets 2 tablespoons olive oil
- ✓ 1 pound chicken tenders, seasoned with kosher salt and fresh ground black pepper
- ✓ 1 egg
- ✓ 1/2 cup panko or gluten-free panko breadcrumbs
- ✓ 1/2 cup + 1 tablespoon shredded Parmesan cheese
- ✓ 1 teaspoon dried basil, crushed between the palms of your hands
- ✓ 1/2 teaspoon dried oregano, crushed between the palms of your hands
- ✓ 1/2 teaspoon dried parsley, crushed between the palms of your hands
- ✓ 1/4 teaspoon granulated garlic
- ✓ 1/4 teaspoon granulated onion
- ✓ Fresh ground black pepper to tast

DIRECTIONS

- ➤ Preheat oven to 425° F. and line a rimmed sheet pan with foil
- ➤ Add the broccoli to the sheet pan
- ➤ Drizzle with the olive oil, sprinkle with salt and pepper and toss to coat.
- ➤ In a resealable freezer bag add the panko, 1/2 cup Parmesan cheese and spices
- ➤ Seal the bag and shake to combine.
- ➤ In a shallow dish whisk together the egg with a tablespoon of water or milk.
- ➤ Add the seasoned chicken tenders to the dish
- ➤ Coat them in the egg mixture. Remove the chicken from the dish and into the freezer bag
- ➤ Shake to coat them in the panko mixture.
- ➤ Place the chicken tenders onto the sheet pan and place it into the oven
- ➤ Bake for 10 minutes then flip the chicken and broccoli over
- ➤ Bake for another 8-10 minutes or until the chicken is cooked through
- ➤ Remove from the oven and sprinkle the broccoli with the remaining tablespoon of Parmesan cheese
- ➤ Serve as is, with a side of marinara sauce or over pasta.

249. MAN CATCHING CHICKEN

Servings: 4 **Cook Time: 50 Min** **Prep Time 40 Min**

INGREDIENTS

- ✓ 4-6 boneless skinless chicken breasts
- ✓ 1/2 cup of Dijon mustard
- ✓ 3/4 cup of maple syrup
- ✓ 1 Tablespoon of red wine vinegar
- ✓ 1 teaspoon of dried rosemary

DIRECTIONS

- ➤ Preheat your oven to 450 degrees.
- ➤ In a small bowl mix together your Dijon mustard, maple syrup, and red wine vinegar.
- ➤ Place your chicken in a sprayed 9 by 13 pan
- ➤ Pour your sauce on top of the chicken
- ➤ Sprinkle with dried Rosemary. Place it uncovered in your preheated oven.
- ➤ Let it bake for 20 minutes and then take them out and flip them over.
- ➤ Cook for another 20 minutes or until your chicken is browned and cooked through.
- ➤ Let the chicken cool for 5 minutes before serving
- ➤ Spoon some extra sauce over the top when you put it on plates.

250. SKINNY CAJUN-STYLE SHRIMP AND GRITS

Servings: 4   **Cook Time: 20 Min**   **Prep Time 10 Min**

INGREDIENTS

CAJUN SEASONING:
- ✓ 1/4 tsp cayenne (plus extra if you really like it spicy!)
- ✓ 1/2 Tbs paprika
- ✓ 2 tsp garlic powder
- ✓ 3/4 tsp freshly cracked black pepper
- ✓ 2 tsp onion powder

ASPARAGUS:
- ✓ 1 1/2 - 2 pounds of asparagus, trimmed
- ✓ Olive oil or coconut oil cooking spray
- ✓ Salt and pepper, to taste
- ✓ 1 lemon, zested and cut into wedges
- ✓ Grits

SAUCY CAJUN SHRIMP:
- ✓ 1 lb jumbo shrimp (medium works too and is often cheaper), peeled and deveined
- ✓ 1/4 cup chopped green onions (greens only)

- ✓ 1 tsp dried oregano
- ✓ 1 tsp dried thyme
- ✓ 1/2 tsp salt
- ✓ 1/2 Tbs whole wheat pastry flour (or regular whole wheat flour)

- ✓ 3 cups water
- ✓ 3/4 cup dry instant grits, plain
- ✓ 1/2 tsp salt
- ✓ 2/3 cup extra sharp cheddar cheese, shredded

- ✓ 1/4 cup low-fat milk
- ✓ Cajun seasoning from above

DIRECTIONS

- ➢ Mix together all of the Cajun seasoning ingredients together in a small bowl and set aside.
- ➢ Heat three cups of water and 3/4 tsp salt in a medium pot to bring to a boil
- ➢ Preheat your oven to 425 degrees.
- ➢ Meanwhile, lay a piece of aluminum foil on a baking sheet
- ➢ Give it a light spray with the olive oil or coconut oil spray
- ➢ Add your trimmed asparagus and give this a quick spray also
- ➢ Next, lightly season with salt, pepper and all of the lemon zest
- ➢ Use your hands to distribute evenly keeping the asparagus in one layer
- ➢ Roast for 5-7 minutes until bright green and cooked through
- ➢ Remove from oven, tent with a piece of foil to keep warm and set aside.

- ➢ Once your pot of water comes to a boil, you can slowly stir in the 3/4 cup of grits
- ➢ Turn the heat down to low, cover and continue to cook for 5-6 minutes
- ➢ (Until thick, stirring once or twice while cooking)
- ➢ Remove from heat and stir in the 2/3 cup of cheese. Cover to keep warm.
- ➢ Season the shrimp well with the Cajun seasoning
- ➢ Heat a large pan to medium and spray with cooking spray
- ➢ Then shrimp to the pan and cook, turning the shrimp once for even cooking
- ➢ Once shrimp are firm and opaque, stir in the 1/4 of milk until thickened
- ➢ (this will happen pretty quickly)
- ➢ Turn off the heat and serve the saucy shrimp immediately with the grits, asparagus
- ➢ Then lemon wedges, sprinkling the chopped green onions over each dish

251. TRADITIONAL RATATOUILLE RECIPE

Servings: 10　　　　　**Cook Time: 30 Min**　　　　　**Prep Time 10 Min**

INGREDIENTS

- ✓ 1 pound eggplant, cut into
- ✓ 1/4 inch circles
- ✓ 2 teaspoons kosher salt
- ✓ 1 tablespoon olive oil
- ✓ 3 cloves garlic, minced
- ✓ 1 teaspoon black pepper
- ✓ 1/4 cup fresh basil, chopped
- ✓ 3/4 cup fresh parsley, chopped
- ✓ 1 large yellow onion, thinly sliced
- ✓ 3 bell peppers (any color), chopped small

- ✓ 1/3 cup dry white wine such as a chardonnay (or substitute vegetable broth)
- ✓ 2 cups no-sugar added tomato sauce
- ✓ 2 large zucchini cut into
- ✓ 1/4 inch circles
- ✓ 2 large yellow squash cut into
- ✓ 1/4 inch circles
- ✓ 4 large tomatoes, peeled and cut into
- ✓ 1/4 inch circles

DIRECTIONS

- ➢ Preheat oven to 400 degrees.
- ➢ Spray a 9 x 13 inch casserole dish with nonstick spray and set aside.
- ➢ Lay the eggplant on a paper towel
- ➢ Sprinkle with half the salt and set aside.
- ➢ Heat the olive oil in a large skillet
- ➢ Add the garlic, half the black pepper, basil, parsley, onion, and bell pepper
- ➢ Cook until the vegetables are soft and add the white wine
- ➢ Simmer for one minute
- ➢ Then add the tomato sauce. Bring to a simmer and remove from heat.
- ➢ Pour half of the sauce into the casserole dish.

- ➢ On top of the sauce place one piece of eggplant, one piece of zucchini
- ➢ Add one piece of yellow squash, and one piece of tomato
- ➢ (Each slightly over lapping).
- ➢ Repeat in long lines over the sauce
- ➢ Spread the remaining sauce over the layer of vegetables
- ➢ Repeat the strips of over lapping eggplant, zucchini, squash, and tomato
- ➢ Sprinkle with remaining salt and black pepper.
- ➢ Bake for 15 to 20 minutes
- ➢ (Or until the vegetables are soft and the top lightly begins to brown)
- ➢ Let cool slightly before serving.

252. FIESTA CHICKEN PASTA BAKE

Servings: 2　　　　　**Cook Time: 40 Min**　　　　　**Prep Time 10 Min**

INGREDIENTS

- ✓ 8 ounces fusili pasta , uncooked (can also use any other pasta shape)
- ✓ 1 cup thick and chunky salsa
- ✓ 1 cup sour cream
- ✓ 1 tablespoon Old El Paso taco seasoning

- ✓ 1 (15 ounce) can whole kernel corn, drained
- ✓ 1 (15 ounce) can black beans, drained and rinsed
- ✓ 2 cups cooked and shredded chicken (rotisserie chicken works well here)

- ✓ 2 cups shredded Monterey Jack and Cheddar cheese , divided (or use all cheddar)
- ✓ (Optional) cilantro or sliced green onions for garnish

DIRECTIONS

- ➢ Cook pasta al dente according to package instructions
- ➢ Will yield about 4 cups cooked pasta. Drain and cool.
- ➢ Preheat oven to 350 degrees. In a large bowl stir together the salsa, sour cream, and taco seasoning
- ➢ Add the cooked pasta and stir to coat.

- ➢ Add the corn, black beans, chicken, and 1 cup of the cheese
- ➢ Toss to combine and pour into a 9x13 baking dish
- ➢ Sprinkle remaining 1 cup of cheese on top.
- ➢ Cover with foil and bake for 20 minutes
- ➢ Take off foil and bake for an additional 5-10 minutes or until cheese is bubbly. Serve

253.   PEANUT NOODLES

Servings: 2   **Cook Time: 30 Min**   **Prep Time 10 Min**

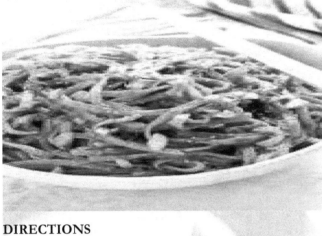

INGREDIENTS
- ✓ 8 ounces spaghetti
- ✓ 2 tablespoons toasted sesame oil
- ✓ 1 bunch green onions, sliced (white parts only - reserve green parts for garnish)
- ✓ 1 teaspoon minced fresh ginger (see Note)
- ✓ 1/3 cup creamy peanut butter (use crunchy if you want nuts in it)
- ✓ 1/4 cup low-sodium soy sauce
- ✓ 1/4 cup hot water
- ✓ 1 Tablespoon cider vinegar
- ✓ 1 teaspoon sugar
- ✓ 1/4 teaspoon crushed red pepper flakes

DIRECTIONS
- ➢ Cook spaghetti in a large pot of salted boiling water until al dente. Drain.
- ➢ While noodles are cooking, prepare the sauce
- ➢ In a small skillet, heat sesame oil over low heat
- ➢ Add the onions (white parts only)
- ➢ Cook until tender. Add the ginger and cook for about 1 minute.
- ➢ Increase the heat to medium
- ➢ Stir in the peanut butter, soy sauce, water, vinegar, sugar, and pepper
- ➢ Stir until combined
- ➢ Remove from heat.
- ➢ Toss spaghetti with sauce, Garnish with sliced green onions and peanuts if desired

RECIPE NOTES: *Fresh ginger can be frozen until ready to use. I don't use a lot of ginger so this is a trick I use often

254. _BAKED SALMON WITH CHORIZO RICE_

Servings: 2 **Cook Time: 45 Min** **Prep Time 10 Min**

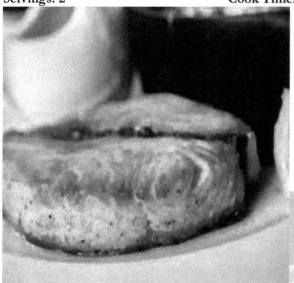

INGREDIENTS:

FOR THE CHORIZO RICE
- ✓ 100g/3½oz chorizo
- ✓ 1 onion, sliced
- ✓ 1 garlic clove, sliced
- ✓ 200g/7oz arborio rice
- ✓ 4 tomatoes, roughly chopped
- ✓ 50g/2oz butter
- ✓ 1 tbsp parsley
- ✓ 600ml/20fl oz chicken stock
- ✓ salt and freshly ground black pepper

FOR THE SALMON
- ➢ 4 x 150g/5oz salmon fillets, skinned
- ➢ 250g/9oz smoked salmon
- ➢ 1 lemon, juice only

DIRECTIONS:

- ➢ Preheat the oven to 180C/350F/Gas 4.
- ➢ Heat a heavy-based frying pan over a medium heat and fry the chorizo for 3-4 minutes, or until crisp
- ➢ Remove the chorizo from the pan with a slotted spoon and set aside.
- ➢ Fry the onion and garlic in the remaining oil for 3-4 minutes, or until soft.
- ➢ Place the chorizo, onion, garlic, rice, tomatoes, butter and parsley into a well-buttered casserole dish
- ➢ Season with salt and freshly ground black pepper.
- ➢ Pour over the chicken stock, cover with a tight-fitting lid
- ➢ Bake in the oven for about 25-30 minutes, or until the rice is cooked.
- ➢ Meanwhile, wrap each salmon fillet in smoked salmon
- ➢ Trim off any excess flesh
- ➢ Season with salt and freshly ground black pepper
- ➢ Squeeze over with the lemon juice.
- ➢ Roast the salmon pieces in the oven for 6-8 minutes, or until cooked through.
- ➢ Serve the salmon on top of the chorizo rice.

255. WARM CRISPY SALMON SALAD

Servings: 2   **Cook Time: 20 Min**   **Prep Time 10 Min**

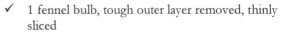

INGREDIENTS:

- ✓ 1 fennel bulb, tough outer layer removed, thinly sliced
- ✓ 8 asparagus spears, trimmed of woody ends and finely shaved with a vegetable peeler or mandoline
- ✓ 8 radishes, thinly sliced
- ✓ 4 salmon fillets, skin on, about 180g/6oz each
- ✓ 30g/1oz plain flour, for dusting
- ✓ 1 tbsp olive oil
- ✓ 250g/9oz Tenderstem broccoli
- ✓ 250g/9oz fine green beans, trimmed
- ✓ 1 tbsp extra virgin olive oil
- ✓ 200g/7oz frozen peas
- ✓ salt and freshly ground black pepper

FOR THE DRESSING
- ✓ 4 tbsp extra virgin olive oil
- ✓ 1 tsp Dijon mustard
- ✓ 1 lemon, juice only
- ✓ 2 tbsp roughly chopped dill

DIRECTIONS:

- ➢ Put the fennel, asparagus and radishes into a bowl of cold water with a handful of ice added
- ➢ Leave to crisp up for 10 minutes or so.
- ➢ Season each salmon fillet with salt and pepper and dust both sides with flour. Heat the olive oil in a large non-stick frying pan over a medium-high heat. Place the salmon skin-side down in the pan
- ➢ Hold down with a spatula for 30 seconds or so
- ➢ Cook, without moving, for 7–8 minutes.
- ➢ Meanwhile, put the broccoli and beans into a sauté pan with 200ml/7fl oz of cold water and extra virgin oil
- ➢ Season well with salt and pepper
- ➢ Bring to the boil and cook over a medium heat
- ➢ Move the veg around so it cooks evenly
- ➢ When the liquid has almost all evaporated, add the frozen peas

- ➢ Once the peas are cooked, remove from the heat and drain off any excess water.
- ➢ When you can see that the skin on the fish is crisp, flip the salmon fillets over
- ➢ Cook for 2 minutes on the other side
- ➢ Remove from the heat and leave to rest while you make the dressing.
- ➢ Whisk the dressing ingredients together in a bowl and pour over the warm veg in the pan
- ➢ Drain the fennel, asparagus and radishes and add to them the pan
- ➢ Toss to mix and season with salt and pepper to taste.
- ➢ Divide the warm salad between serving plates
- ➢ Top each portion with a salmon fillet, crisped skin side up, to serve.

Servings: 2   **Cook Time: 20 Min**   **Prep Time 10 Min**

INGREDIENTS:

- ✓ 200g/7oz Puy lentils
- ✓ 1 bay leaf
- ✓ 200g/7oz fine green beans, chopped
- ✓ 25g/1oz flat leaf parsley, chopped
- ✓ 2 tbsp Dijon mustard
- ✓ 2 tbsp capers, rinsed and chopped

- ✓ 2 tbsp olive oil
- ✓ 2 lemons, finely sliced
- ✓ Salmon fillets, about 500g/1lb 2oz in total
- ✓ 1 fennel bulb, finely sliced
- ✓ Fill sprigs, to garnish
- ✓ Salt and freshly ground black pepper

DIRECTIONS:

- ➤ Put the lentils in a saucepan with the bay leaf and enough cold water to cover
- ➤ Bring to the boil, reduce to a simmer
- ➤ Cook for 30 minutes or until tender
- ➤ Season to taste with salt and freshly ground black pepper
- ➤ Add the beans and simmer for a further minute.
- ➤ Drain the lentils and discard the bay leaf
- ➤ Stir in the parsley, mustard, capers and oil.

- ➤ Preheat the grill to a hot setting.
- ➤ Arrange the lemon slices on a foil-lined grill pan
- ➤ Place the salmon and fennel slices on top
- ➤ Season the salmon and fennel with salt and freshly ground black pepper
- ➤ Cook under the grill for about 10 minutes, or until the salmon is cooked through.
  Place the salmon on top of the lentils and fennel slices, garnish with dill sprigs and serve

257. SHRIMP WITH BREADCRUMB PASTA

Servings: 4 **Cook Time: 25Min** **Prep Time 10 Min**

INGREDIENTS

FOR THE BREADCRUMBS
- ✓ 1 tablespoon unsalted butter
- ✓ 1/2 cup Panko breadcrumbs
- ✓ 1/8 teaspoon kosher salt
- ✓ 1/8 teaspoon freshly ground black pepper

PINCH CAYENNE PEPPER
- ✓ 1/8 teaspoon garlic powder For the Shrimp Pasta
- ✓ 1/2 cup whole-milk plain Greek yogurt
- ✓ 2 tablespoons Asian chili-garlic sauce
- ✓ 1/2 teaspoon honey
- ✓ 1/4 teaspoon garlic powder
- ✓ 3-4 tablespoons lime juice
- ✓ 12 ounces dry spaghetti
- ✓ 1 pound uncooked peeled and deveined medium shrimp
- ✓ 1/2 teaspoon kosher salt, plus more for the pasta water
- ✓ 1/8 teaspoon black pepper. more to taste
- ✓ 1/8 teaspoon cayenne pepper
- ✓ 2 medium scallions, thinly sliced, divided

DIRECTIONS

- ➢ To make the breadcrumbs, melt the butter in a small skillet over medium heat
- ➢ Add the breadcrumbs, salt, black pepper, cayenne pepper, and garlic powder
- ➢ Cook for 4 minutes or until golden, crispy, and fragrant, stirring constantly. Set aside.
- ➢ To prepare the shrimp pasta
- ➢ Place a rack in the middle of the oven and heat to 400°F
- ➢ Lightly coat a rimmed baking sheet with cooking spray
- ➢ Then set aside.
- ➢ Bring a large pot of salted water to a boil. In the meantime
- ➢ Whisk the yogurt, chili-garlic sauce, honey, garlic powder
- ➢ Add half of the lime juice together in a small bowl; set aside.
- ➢ When the water is boiling
- ➢ Then add the pasta and cook according to package directions.
- ➢ Meanwhile, pat the shrimp dry
- ➢ Place on the prepared baking sheet
- ➢ Season with the salt, black pepper, and cayenne and stir to coat
- ➢ Spread into an even layer.
- ➢ Roast for about 7 minutes or until the shrimp is opaque and pink
- ➢ Stirring halfway through
- ➢ Drizzle the remaining lime juice over the shrimp
- ➢ Toss to coat, scraping up any flavorful bits on the baking sheet.
- ➢ Drain the pasta and return it to the pot
- ➢ Pour in the yogurt sauce and toss to coat the pasta
- ➢ Join also the shrimp and any juices from the baking sheet, along with half of the scallions, and gently toss again
- ➢ Serve sprinkled with the crispy breadcrumbs and remaining scallions.
- ➢ Enjoy!

258. SEA BREEZE SALMON SALAD WITH MARGARITA DRESSING

Servings: 4　　　　　　　**Cook Time: 15Min**　　　　　　**Prep Time 5 Min**

INGREDIENTS

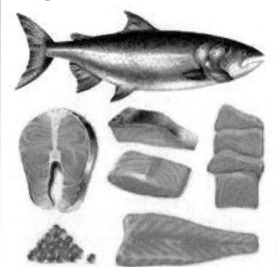

- ✓ 1 pound fresh or frozen salmon fillets, cut into 4 pieces
- ✓ 5 tablespoons extra-virgin olive oil, divided
- ✓ 3 tablespoons freshly squeezed lime juice, divided
- ✓ 2 teaspoons Jamaican jerk seasoning
- ✓ 6 cups tightly packed mixed greens or spring mix lettuce
- ✓ 1 cup fresh strawberries, sliced
- ✓ 1 mango, diced
- ✓ 1 avocado, diced
- ✓ ¼ cup sliced or slivered almonds
- ✓ 1 tablespoon honey
- ✓ 1½ teaspoons ground cumin
- ✓ ⅛ teaspoon salt
- ✓ Fresh cilantro, for garnish

DIRECTIONS

- ➢ Thaw the fish in cold water if using frozen, and preheat the oven to 400°F.
- ➢ Place the fillets on a baking sheet, and brush with 1 tablespoon of olive oil
- ➢ Then drizzle with 1 tablespoon of lime juice
- ➢ Sprinkle with the jerk seasoning
- ➢ Broil the fish on the top rack for 12 to 14 minutes
- ➢ (Or until it reaches an internal temperature of 145°F and the salmon flakes easily with a fork)
- ➢ Remove from the oven and allow to cool.
- ➢ Meanwhile, in a large serving bowl
- ➢ Layer the salad greens followedby the strawberries, mango, avocado, and almonds

- ➢ Toss gently to mix.
- ➢ In a small bowl, prepare the dressing
- ➢ Whisk together the remaining 4 tablespoons of olive oil
- ➢ Add the remaining 2 tablespoons of lime juice
- ➢ Then the honey, cumin, and salt.
- ➢ To serve, arrange the salad mix on 4 plates
- ➢ Top each salad with one salmon fillet, and gently flake apart
- ➢ Add the dressing, and garnish with fresh cilantro, if desired

Servings: 4   **Cook Time: 20Min**   **Prep Time 5 Min**

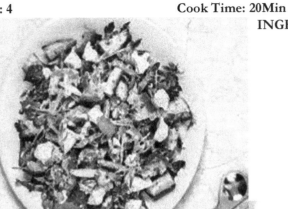

INGREDIENTS

- ✓ ½ pound precooked frozen shrimp
- ✓ 3 slices day-old French or sourdough bread, cut into bite-size cubes
- ✓ 10 medium asparagus spears
- ✓ 6 cups loosely packed fresh spinach
- ✓ 4 Roma tomatoes, quartered or sliced
- ✓ ½ red onion, thinly sliced
- ✓ 4 tablespoons extra-virgin olive oil
- ✓ 2 tablespoons balsamic vinegar Pinch salt
- ✓ 1 avocado, diced
- ✓ About 5 large fresh basil leaves
- ✓ ½ cup shredded Parmesan cheese

DIRECTIONS

- ➢ Thaw the shrimp by placing in a large bowl of cold water
- ➢ Preheat the oven to 300°F.
- ➢ Arrange the bread on a baking sheet in a single layer
  Toast until it becomes crunchy, 5 to 10 minutes total, flipping once during baking.
- ➢ Meanwhile, on a second baking sheet
  Arrange the asparagus in a single layer
- ➢ After removing the bread, raise the oven temperature to 375°F
- ➢ Roast the asparagus until it's a vibrant green color and is cooked through

- ➢ (About 10 minutes)
- ➢ In a salad bowl toss the spinach with the tomatoes
- ➢ Add onion, olive oil vinegar, and salt.
- ➢ Add the avocado to the salad
- ➢ Once the asparagus is roasted, cut into 1- to 2-inch pieces
- ➢ Add to the bowl. Mix to combine
- ➢ Then peel the shrimp and add to the salad
- ➢ Top with the toasted bread. Toss one last time
- ➢ Then transfer to four bowls or plates
- ➢ Chiffonade the basil (see tip)
- ➢ Garnish with the basil and Parmesan cheese, and serve

CONCLUSION

The hectic everyday life, planned and sudden professional commitments, prevent you from following a correct and healthy diet. This book contains typical recipes from the Busy Man Diet. Using the recipes in this book as a reference, you will be able to organise a dietary plan that is appropriate for your busy schedule and to have a healthy diet as well as lose excess weight. The book contains recipes for all budgets so you will have no trouble shopping. Have fun and enjoy your diet!

Thanks for reading this book